VACCINATION AND CONTROL OF AUJESZKY'S DISEASE

Current Topics in Veterinary Medicine and Animal Science

Recent publications

1984

26. Manipulation of Growth in Farm Animals, edited by J.F. Roche and D. O'Callaghan. ISBN 0–89838–617–8
27. Latent Herpes Virus Infections in Veterinary Medicine, edited by G. Wittmann, R.M. Gaskell and H.-J. Rziha. ISBN 0–89838–622–5
28. Grassland Beef Production, edited by W. Holmes. ISBN 0–89838–650–0
29. Recent Advances in Virus Diagnosis, edited by M.S. McNulty and J.B. McFerran. ISBN 0–89838–674–8
30. The Male in Farm Animal Reproduction, edited by M. Courot. ISBN 0–89838–682–9

1985

31. Endocrine Causes of Seasonal and Lactational Anestrus in Farm Animals, edited by F. Ellendorff and F. Elsaesser. ISBN 0–89838–738–8
32. Brucella Melitensis, edited by J.M. Verger and M. Plommet. ISBN 0–89838–742–6

1986

33. Diagnosis of Mycotoxicoses, edited by J.L. Richard and J.R. Thurston. ISBN 0–89838–751–5
34. Embryonic Mortality in Farm Animals, edited by J.M. Sreenan and M.G. Diskin. ISBN 0–89838–772–8
35. Social Space for Domestic Animals, edited by R. Zayan. ISBN 0–89838–773–6
36. The Present State of Leptospirosis Diagnosis and Control, edited by W.A. Ellis and T.W.A. Little. ISBN 0–89838–777–9
37. Acute Virus Infections of Poultry, edited by J.B. McFerran and M.S. McNulty. ISBN 0–89838–809–0

1987

38. Evaluation and Control of Meat Quality in Pigs, edited by P.V. Tarrant, G. Eikelenboom and G. Monin. ISBN 0–89838–854–6
39. Follicular Growth and Ovulation Rate in Farm Animals, edited by J.F. Roche and D. O'Callaghan. ISBN 0–89838–855–4
40. Cattle Housing Systems, Lameness and Behaviour, edited by H.K. Wierenga and D.J. Peterse. ISBN 0–89838–862–7
41. Physiological and Pharmacological Aspects of the Reticulo-rumen, edited by L.A.A. Ooms, A.D. Degryse and A.S.J.P.A.M. van Miert. ISBN 0–89838–878–3
42. Biology of Stress in Farm Animals: An Integrative Approach, edited by P.R. Wiepkema and P.W.M. van Adrichem. ISBN 0–89838–895–3
43. Helminth Zoonoses, edited by S. Geerts, V. Kumar and J. Brandt. ISBN 0–89838–896–1
44. Energy Metabolism in Farm Animals: Effects of Housing, Stress and Disease, edited by M.W.A. Verstegen and A.M. Henken. ISBN 0–89838–974–7
45. Summer Mastitis, edited by G. Thomas, H.J. Over, U. Vecht and P. Nansen. ISBN 0–89838–982–8

1988

46. Modelling of Livestock Production Systems, edited by S. Korver and J.A.M. van Arendonk. ISBN 0–89838–373–0
47. Increasing Small Ruminant Productivity in Semi-arid Areas, edited by E.F. Thomson and F.S. Thomson. ISBN 0–89838–386–2
48. The Management and Health of Farmed Deer, edited by H.W. Reid. ISBN 0–89838–408–7

1989

49. Vaccination and Control of Aujeszky's Disease, edited by J.T. van Oirschot. ISBN 0–7923–0184–6

Vaccination and Control of Aujeszky's Disease

A Seminar in the Community Programme for the Coordination of Agricultural Research, held at the Berlaymont Building, Brussels, Belgium, 5-6 July 1988

Sponsored by the Commission of the European Communities, Directorate-General for Agriculture, Coordination of Agricultural Research

Edited by

J. T. VAN OIRSCHOT

Department of Virology,
Central Veterinary Institute,
Lelystad, The Netherlands

KLUWER ACADEMIC PUBLISHERS

DORDRECHT / BOSTON / LONDON

FOR THE COMMISSION OF THE EUROPEAN COMMUNITIES

PREFACE

Aujeszky's disease (AD) is a major economic threat to pig industries around the world. England and Denmark have implemented a programme to eradicate AD virus from their territory. Because of the relatively low prevalence of AD in these countries, they have been able to avoid vaccinating pigs against AD. Therefore, their eradication scheme is based on identifying infected pigs by conventional serological methods and slaughtering infected pigs. Other countries of the European Community cannot use such an approach, because of their widespread use of vaccines against AD. The discrepancy between those countries that are free from AD virus and those that are not may in the future hamper the free trade of pigs in Europe. Therefore, the implementing of programmes for the control of AD should be considered in European countries other than England and Denmark. In the United States of America national attention is increasingly being focussed on controlling AD.

The objectives of this meeting were to review recent developments in molecular biology, vaccinology and detection of epitope-specific antibodies to AD virus and to discuss their impact on the control of AD in countries that practise vaccination.

I thank the Directorate-General for Agriculture of the Commission of the European Communities for giving me the opportunity and financial support to organize this seminar. The seminar and the preparation of these proceedings were also made possible by grants from Agritech GmbH, Cyanamid, Duphar BV, IFFA Mérieux, Intervet International BV, The Upjohn Company, Smith-Kline RIT, and Syntrovet.

J.T. van Oirschot

Lelystad, October 1988.

1. DELETION MUTANT VACCINES AGAINST AUJESZKY'S DISEASE

Chairpersons T. Ben-Porat and A.L.J. Gielkens

ANALYSIS OF THE FACTORS THAT AFFECT VIRULENCE OF PSEUDORABIES VIRUS

T.C. Mettenleiter, B. Lomniczi**, L. Zsák**, I. Medveczky**, T. Ben-Porat***, A.S. Kaplan****

*Bundesforschungsanstalt für Viruskrankheiten der Tiere, D-7400 Tübingen, FRG.
**Veterinary Medical Research Institute, Hungarian Academy of Sciences H-1581 Budapest, Hungary
***Department of Microbiology Vanderbilt University School of Medicine Nashville, Tennessee 37232

ABSTRACT

Two complementary approaches have been used to elucidate the viral functions necessary for the expression of virulence of pseudorabies virus (PRV): (1) marker rescue of avirulent strains, thereby identifying the functions that are defective and contribute to avirulence; (2) introduction of mutations within the genes encoding functions nonessential for growth in vitro into wild-type virus and determination of the effect of these mutations on virulence. We describe in this report an analysis of the defects in the Bartha vaccine strain. This strain was shown to be defective in the genes encoding glycoproteins gI, gIII and in a capsid protein. Bartha virus that had been marker rescued with all 3 of these genes derived from PRV (Ka) was virulent; restoration of any one of these genes to the Bartha strain did not restore virulence. Deletion mutants of PRV (Ka) defective in the genes encoding either gI or gIII had a reduced virulence for day-old chickens as well as for swine. The double mutants gI$^-$/gIII$^-$ had completely lost their virulence. The results obtained indicate that several gene products which individually affect virulence only slightly can act synergistically; combinations of defects in these gene products abolish virulence.

INTRODUCTION

Vaccination of swine with attenuated strains of pseudorabies virus (PRV) is practiced in most countries to prevent outbreaks of Aujeszky's disease. Several attenuated strains have been isolated by repeated passage in cell culture. These attenuated strains do not cause disease in swine and provide varying degrees of immunity against superinfection with virulent strains (Gustafson, 1975).

PRV has a large genome that may encode as many as 100 proteins. The proteins that are defective in the avirulent strains have, for the most part, not been identified.

J. T. van Oirschot (ed.), Vaccination and Control of Aujeszky's Disease, 3–11.

To elucidate the functions necessary for the expression of virulence of PRV, studies designed to uncover the genetic basis of the avirulence of these strains have been undertaken. Two complementary approaches have been used: (1) marker rescue of avirulent strains, thereby attempting to identify the functions that are defective in these strains; (2) introduction into wild-type virus of mutations within the genes encoding functions nonessential for growth in vitro and determination of the effect of these mutations on virulence.

Previous studies have led to the conclusions that defects in several loci of the PRV genome may affect virulence without necessarily affecting virus growth in cell culture (Lomniczi *et al.*, 1984b; 1987a; 1987b). Furthermore, it has been shown that most vaccine strains have multiple defects contributing to their lack of virulence, with the exception of the Tatarov strain which appears to only have a defect in the thymidine kinase (TK) gene (Lomniczi *et al.*, 1987a).

In this report we summarize some of our results relating to the functions required for the expression of virulence. Some of these results deal with the analysis of the defects in 1 vaccine strain, the Bartha strain, to which virulence has been restored by marker rescue. Others deal with the virulence of mutants of PRV that have been rendered defective in nonessential viral glycoproteins.

RESULTS AND DISCUSSION

Identification of defects in the Bartha strain that contribute to its loss of virulence

The Bartha vaccine strain has a deletion in the unique short (U_S) component (Lomniczi *et al.*, 1984a; Berns *et al.*,1985) which spans the sequences encoding glycoproteins gI, gp63 and an 11K protein (Mettenleiter *et al.*, 1985; Petrovskis et al., 1986; Petrovskis and Post, 1987). An intact U_S component (R1, see Fig. 1) was introduced into Bartha 43/25a, thereby restoring to the virus the ability to synthesize these proteins (Lomniczi *et al.*, 1987b). Bartha 43/25a is not virulent (Table 1). After further marker rescue of Bartha 43/25a with another sequence wild-type DNA, Bam HI fragment 4 (R2, see Fig. 1), a sequence that encodes 4 capsid proteins (Lomniczi *et al.*, 1987b), the variant Bartha 43/25aB4 that was obtained was partially virulent. Deletion of gI from Bartha 43/25aB4 renders it avirulent (Table 1), indicating that gI is of importance in the restoration of virulence by the sequences in the U_S (Mettenleiter *et al.*, 1987b).

The Bartha strain and its derivatives encode a gIII ($gIII^B$) glycoprotein that is atypical and differs in several respects from wild-type PRV(Ka). Because gIII affects virulence of PRV(Ka) (see below), we considered the possibility that the "atypical" gIII^B contributes to the lack of virulence of the Bartha strain. The resident gIII^B gene was therefore replaced with the gIII gene of PRV(Ka) (R3), as described in detail elsewhere (Mettenleiter *et al.*, 1988b).

The results in Table 1 show that whereas there was no significant difference between the titers of infectious virus produced by cells infected with the different Bartha variants, the differences in their virulence for day-old chickens inoculated intracerebrally was considerable. Bartha and Bartha 43/25a were avirulent and the doubly rescued Bartha 43/25aB4 had a low level of virulence. After acquisition of gIII^{Ka}, 43/25aB4 became 15 to 20-fold more virulent. Thus, the resident gIII^B gene in the Bartha strain was defective and this defect contributed to the low level of virulence of Bartha 43/25aB4.

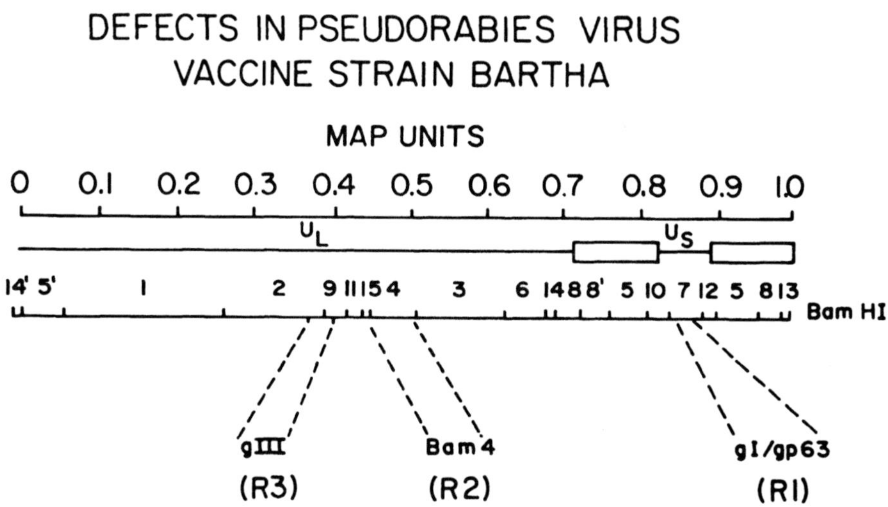

Fig. 1 The regions of the genome that have been marker rescued to restore virulence (R1), (R2) and (R3) are indicated (see text for details).

Table 1 also shows that Bartha and Bartha 43/25a were avirulent for swine; Bartha 43/25aB4 had acquired some virulence; Bartha 43/25aB4-gIII^{Ka} killed all the animals, as did wild-type PRV(Ka). Thus, the LD50 for day-old chickens of the various virus variants paralleled their virulence for 3-week-old pigs, i.e., a good correlation between virulence of PRV variants for day-old chickens and for swine exists.

We conclude from the results described above that the Bartha strain is defective in at least 3 genes affecting virulence; gI, gIII, and a capsid protein that is encoded in Bam HI fragment 4. Restoration of either gI or of a functional gIII only, as well as restoration of both gI and gIII to the Bartha strain, does not restore its virulence (Table 1, and Mettenleiter *et al.*, 1988b); restoration of a functional Bam HI fragment 4 also does not restore virulence (Lomniczi *et al.*, 1987b). However, restoration of Bam HI fragment 4 and an intact U_S (i.e., glycoprotein gI) restores partial virulence. Restoration of all 3 functions to the Bartha strain (i.e., Bam HI fragment 4, an intact U_S and substitution of $gIII^{Ka}$ for $gIII^{B}$) results in a variant that has a level of virulence that is only slightly lower than that of wild-type virus (Table 1).

TABLE 1 Virulence of different marker rescued Bartha variants

Bartha variants	Virus genotype	Virus yield[a] (PFU/cell)	Virulence: Chickens[b]	Pigs[c] Expt. 1	Pigs[c] Expt.2
Bartha	$gI^-/gp63^-/B4^-$[d]$/gIII^B$[e]	210	$>10^6$	0/5	0/5
Bartha $gIII^{Ka}$	$gI^-/gp63^-/B4^-/gIII^{Ka}$[f]	250	$>10^6$	0/5	ND
Bartha 43/25a	$gI^+/gp63^+/B4^-/gIII^B$	220	$>10^6$	0/5	0/5
Bartha 43/25a-$gIII^{Ka}$	$gI^+/gp63^+/B4^-/gIII^{Ka}$	230	$>10^6$	0/5	ND
Bartha 43/25aB4$^+$	$gI^+/gp63^+/B4^+/gIII^B$	250	$1x10^4$	4/5	2/5
Bartha 43/25aB4$^+$gI$^-$	$gI^-/gp63^+/B4^+/gIII^B$	230	$>10^6$	ND	ND
Bartha 43/25aB4$^+$$gIII^{Ka}$	$gI^+/gp63^+/B4^+/gIII^{Ka}$	240	$7x10^2$	5/5	ND
Wild-type PRV(Ka)		270	$5x10^1$	5/5	5/5

[a] PK cells were infected (5 PFU/cell) and incubated for 48 h in Eagles medium containing 5% dialyzed calf serum and the virus yield was determined.
[b] The LD_{50} was determined by the Reed and Muench method (1938).
[c] Three-week-old pigs were inoculated both intranasally and intramuscularly with 10^7 PFU each of either wild-type or mutant virus. The animals were observed for 14 days. Animals exhibiting severe nervous signs were sacrificed. Nominator, animals that showed severe signs of disease; denominator, number of animals inoculated.
[d] The variants of Bartha that were marker-rescued with Bam HI fragment 4 are indicated by a B4$^+$; those that were not marker-rescued are indicated by a B4$^-$.
[e] $gIII^B$ denotes the resident Bartha glycoprotein gIII gene.
[f] $gIII^{Ka}$ denotes the PRV(Ka) gIII gene.

Virulence of mutants of PRV(Ka) defective in the expression of glycoproteins gI, gp63, gIII or a combination thereof

Glycoproteins gI, gp63, and gIII are nonessential for growth of PRV in cell culture (Ben-Porat *et al.*, 1986; Mettenleiter *et al.*, 1985; Petrovskis *et al.*, 1986; Robbins *et al.*, 1986; Wathen and Wathen, 1986). Mutants of wild-type PRV(Ka) defective in the expression of these glycoproteins were constructed (Mettenleiter *et al.*, 1987a; 1988b). Fig. 2 illustrates the deletions introduced into the PRV(Ka) genome to inactivate the genes encoding these glycoproteins.

The ability of the various mutants to grow in cultures of RK cells, their ability to kill day-old chickens when inoculated intracerebrally (IC), as well as their virulence for pigs, was determined (Table 2). Mutants of PRV defective in either gI ($gIII^+/gI^-/gp63^+$), or defective in both gI and gp63 ($gIII^+/gI^-/gp63^-$), grow as well as wild-type virus in cell culture and have only a slightly increased LD_{50} for chickens. They also are somewhat less virulent for pigs than is wild-type virus (Mettenleiter *et al.*, 1987b). Mutants defective in gIII ($gIII^-/gI^+/gp63^+$) yielded only approximately 25% as many PFU as did cultures infected with wild-type virus. The reduction in titer of infectious virus obtained from $gIII^-$ virus-infected cultures is due, in large part, to a less effective and slower rate of adsorption of the $gIII^-$ mutants to its host cells, thereby reducing the number of PFU obtained (Schreurs *et al.*, 1988). Despite the lower yield of PFU obtained from cells infected with the $gIII^-$ mutant, the LD_{50} of this mutant for chickens was only somewhat lower than that of PRV(Ka) virus (Table 2). Its virulence for pigs appeared, however, to be decreased more significantly.

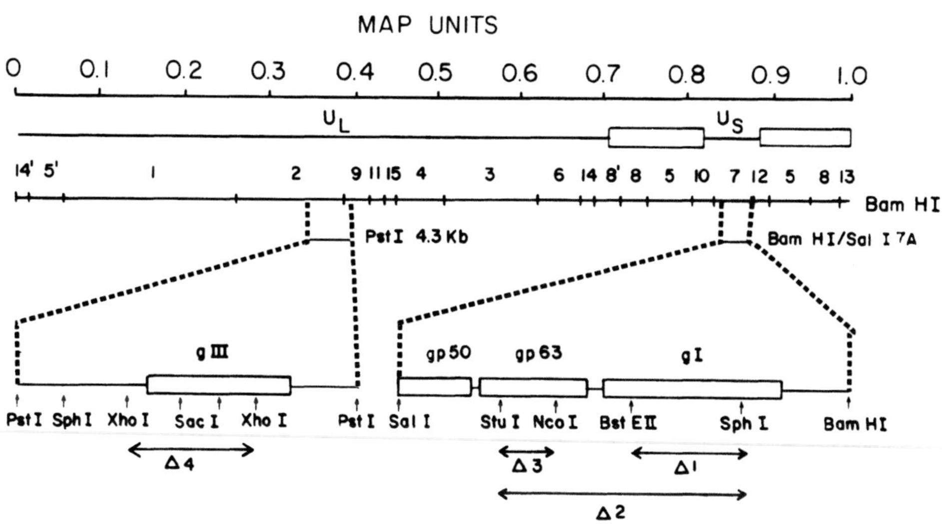

Fig.2 Map of PRV mutants with deletions in the genes encoding gI (Δ1), gI/gp63 (Δ2), gp63 (Δ3) or gIII (Δ4). The top of the figure shows the Bam HI restriction map of PRV DNA. The positions of the genes are shown on line 4. The sequences in the genes that span the deletions are indicated by the arrows.

Cells infected with the double mutants $gIII^-/gI^-$ ($gIII^-/gI^-gp63^+$), or the triple mutant $gIII^-/gI^-/gp63^-$ yielded only a slightly lower titer of infectious virus (about 2-3 fold lower) than did cells infected with mutants defective in gIII alone. However, in contrast to the mutants defective in either gIII or gI, which were only slightly less virulent than wild-type virus for chickens, the double or triple mutants were completely avirulent for chickens; they were completely avirulent for pigs as well (Table 2). Again, it is worthy to note that there is a relatively good correlation between the effects of inactivation of a given gene on the virulence of the mutant for chickens and for swine, i.e., day-old chickens are a relatively good model system in which to test virulence of PRV.

TABLE 2 Growth and virulence of deletion mutants of PRV(Ka) defective in the synthesis of different glycoproteins

Virus genotype	Virus yield (PFU/cell)	Virulence Chickens (LD50)	Pigs Expt.1	Pigs Expt.2
$gIII^+/gI^+/gp63^+$	220	$< 1x10^2$	5/5	4/5
$gIII^+/gI^-/gp63^+\Delta$	190	$2x10^2$	2/5	ND
$gIII^+/gI^-/gp63^-\Delta$	170	$2x10^2$	2/5	ND
$gIII^-/gI^+/gp63^+\Delta$	54	$2x10^2$	ND	1/5
$gIII^-/gI^-/gp63^+\Delta$	23	$> 10^5$	ND	0/5
$gIII^-/gI^-/gp63^-\Delta$	33	$> 10^5$	ND	0/5
$gIII^-/gI^+/gp63^+$MAR-M7pl	78	$2x10^2$	1/5	ND

Δ denotes deletion mutant; MAR-M7pl denotes a monoclonal-resistant mutant that does not express gIII (Ben-Porat *et al.*, 1986).
ND, not determined. See legend to Table 1 for experimental details.

The results obtained with the deletion mutants of PRV(Ka) show that gI, as well as gIII, play a role in virulence but that the effect of the deletion of one of these glycoproteins is marked especially when it occurs in conjunction with the deletion of the other. In chickens, the effect of a deletion of gI on virulence clearly appears to be synergistic with a deletion of gIII. The LD_{50}s of the virus in pigs were not determined because of the expense involved and it is not possible from the data available to ascertain whether in this case also inactivation of gI and gIII have a synergistic effect on virulence. It is clear, however, that (1) viruses defective in either gI or gIII are less virulent for swine than viruses that express these glycoproteins. (2) The double mutants $gI^-/gIII^-$ have completely lost virulence for swine. The results obtained with marker rescue of Bartha variants (Table 1) and those obtained with the deletion mutants of PRV(Ka) (Table 2), lead to similar conclusions, i.e., that gI (and gp63), as well as gIII, play a role in virulence.

To understand how these glycoproteins affect virulence, it is necessary to correlate their functions during the interactions of the virus with its host cells, with their functions in the development of disease. Although the glycoproteins, the effects of which we have studied, are nonessential and can be dispensed with for growth in cell culture, a detailed analysis of their interactions with their host cells revealed that they fulfill important functions (Mettenleiter *et al.*, 1987a; Schreurs *et al.*, 1988). Thus, glycoprotein gIII affects adsorption, the earliest event leading to virus replication; in the absence of gIII, the infective process is initiated but occurs more slowly and with a lower efficiency than with wild-type virus (Schreurs *et al.*, 1988). Glycoprotein gIII, as well as gI, also play a role in virus release (Mettenleiter *et al.*, 1987a; Schreurs *et al.*, 1988; Whealy *et al.*, 1988). These observations on the interaction of the deletion mutants with their host cells in vitro indicate possible mechanisms by which the glycoproteins may affect virulence. Adsorption to specific cells plays a pivotal role in cell tropism and pathogenesis. Furthermore, efficient release from the infected cells is an important aspect of virus replication since it promotes the propagation of the virus. Of particular interest is the finding that the effect of gI on virus growth is type-cell specific (Mettenleiter *et al.*, 1988; Zuckermann *et al.*, 1988), i.e., the ability of the virus to be propagated in certain organs (but not in others) may be affected by this glycoprotein.

CONCLUSIONS

Several conclusions regarding the elements that confer virulence upon PRV can be drawn from our studies. (1) Virulence of PRV is determined multigenically. (2) Defects in genes that affect virulence do not necessarily affect in a detectable manner the growth of the virus in cell culture. (3) While several gene products of PRV have been shown to contribute to the expression of virulence, lack of expression of any one of these genes alone (with the exception of the TK gene) does not abolish virulence; it only decreases it. (4) Most vaccine strains are defective in several functions that affect virulence. (5) The nonessential glycoproteins gI and gIII affect virulence and do so synergistically.

The identification of the viral factors involved in virulence does not per se clarify how they contribute to the pathogenesis of the virus and to the development of disease. However, the study of the interactions of mutants in defined proteins with cells in vitro are contributing information which indicates how these proteins may affect the development of disease.

ACKNOWLEDGEMENTS

This investigation was supported by a grant (AI-10947) from the National Institutes of Health. Thomas C. Mettenleiter was supported by a fellowship (Me 854/1-2) from the Deutsche Forschungsgemeinschaft.

REFERENCES

Ben-Porat, T., DeMarchi, J.M., Lomniczi, B. and Kaplan, A.S. 1986. Role of glycoproteins of pseudorabies virus in eliciting neutralizing antibodies. Virol., **154**, 325-334.

Berns, A., Van der Ouweland, A., Quint, W., Van Oirschot, J.T. and Gielkens, A. 1985. Presence of markers for virulence in the unique short region or repeat region or both of pseudorabies hybrid viruses. J. Virol., **53**, 89-93.

Gustafson, D.P. 1975. Pseudorabies. In "Disease of Swine". Fourth Edition (Ed. H.D. Dunne and A.D. Leman). (Iowa State University Press, Ames, Iowa). pp. 391-410.

Lomniczi, B., Blankenship, M.L. and Ben-Porat, T. 1984a. Deletions in the genome of pseudorabies vaccine strains and existence of four isomeric forms. J. Virol., **49**, 970-979.

Lomniczi, B., Kaplan, A.S. and Ben-Porat, T. 1987a. Multiple defects in the genome of pseudorabies virus can affect virulence without detectably affecting replication in cell culture. Virol., **161**, 181-189.

Lomniczi, B., Watanabe, S., Ben-Porat, T. and Kaplan, A.S. 1984b. Genetic basis of the neurovirulence of pseudorabies virus. J. Virol., **52**, 198-205.

Lomniczi, B., Watanabe, S., Ben-Porat, T. and Kaplan, A.S. 1987b. Genome location and identification of functions defective in the Bartha vaccine strain of pseudorabies virus. J. Virol., **61**, 796-801.

Mettenleiter, T.C., Lomniczi, B., Sugg, N., Schreurs, C. and Ben-Porat, T. 1988a. Host cell-specific growth advantage of pseudorabies virus with a deletion in the genome sequences encoding a structural glycoprotein, J. Virol., **62**, 12-19.

Mettenleiter, T.C., Lukacs, N., Rziha, H.J. 1985. Pseudorabies virus avirulent strains fail to express a major glycoprotein. J. Virol., **56**, 307-311.

Mettenleiter, T.C., Schreurs, C., Zuckermann, F. and Ben-Porat, T. 1987a. Role of pseudorabies virus glycoprotein gI in virus release from infected cells. J. Virol., **61**, 2764-2769.

Mettenleiter, T.C., Schreurs, C., Zuckermann, F., Ben-Porat, T. and Kaplan, A.S. 1988b. Role of glycoprotein gIII of pseudorabies virus in virulence. J. Virol., **62**, 2712-2717.

Mettenleiter, T.C., Zsak, L., Kaplan, A.S., Ben-Porat, T. and Lomniczi, B. 1987b. Role of a structural glycoprotein of a herpesvirus (pseudorabies) in virus virulence. J. Virol., **61**, 4030-4032.

Petrovskis, E., Timmins, J.G., Gierman, T.M. and Post, L.E. 1986. Deletions in vaccine strains of pseudorabies virus and their effect on synthesis of glycoprotein gp63. J. Virol., **60**, 1166-1169.

Petrovskis, E. and Post, L.E. 1987. A small open reading frame in PRV and implication for evolutionary relationships between herpesviruses. Virol., **159**, 193-195.

Reed, L.J. and Muench, M. 1938. A simple method of estimating fifty percent end points. Am. J. Hyg., **27**, 493-497.

Robbins, A.K., Whealy, M.E., Watson, R.J. and Enquist, L.W. 1986. The pseudorabies virus gene encoding glycoprotein gIII is not essential for growth in tissue culture. J. Virol., **59**, 635-645.

Schreurs, C., Mettenleiter, T.C., Zuckermann, F., Sugg, N. and Ben-Porat, T. 1988. Glycoprotein gIII of pseudorabies virus is multifunctional. J. Virol., **62**, 2251-2257.

Wathen, M.W. and Wathen, L.M.K. 1986. Characterization and mapping of a nonessential pseudorabies virus glycoprotein. J. Virol., **58**, 173-178.

Whealy, M.E., Robbins, A.K. and Enquist, L.W. 1988. Pseudorabies virus glycoprotein gIII is required for efficient growth in tissue culture. J. Virol., **62**, 2512-2515.

Zuckermann, F.A., Mettenleiter, T.C., Schreurs, C., Sugg, N. and Ben-Porat, T. 1988. Complex between glycoproteins gI and gp63 of pseudorabies virus: Its effect on virus replication. Submitted for publication.

THE USE OF THE gX DELETED VACCINE PRVΔTKΔgX-1 IN THE CONTROL OF AUJESZKY'S DISEASE

R.C. Wardley, L.E. Post

The Upjohn Company
Kalamazoo, Michigan 49001, U.S.A.

ABSTRACT

The worldwide increase in the incidence of pseudorabies since the early 1970's has resulted in an increasing use of vaccines to help control the disease. Most of these vaccines have been conventionally produced gI deleted products and whilst helping control clinical signs, they have overseen a steady rise in the incidence of disease. More recently, gX deleted vaccines have become available and this paper deals with how well gX deleted vaccines perform in the 3 crucial areas of preventing challenge virus shedding, latency and in sow/piglet usage programs. In comparative trials animals vaccinated with the deletion vaccine PRVΔtkΔgX-1 (Tolvid) and challenged with field virus lost less weight than pigs vaccinated with 2 conventionally deleted gI-negative vaccines. Furthermore, Tolvid appears to reduce latency, a factor thought by many epidemiologists to be crucial if pseudorabies is to be successfully controlled. A further major problem with pseudorabies virus vaccination programs is that passive immunity interferes with vaccination and hence piglets can be vaccinated and thought to be protected, whereas the vaccine has not "taken" and the piglet remains vulnerable to infection. To test the use of Tolvid in this situation piglets born to Tolvid vaccinated sows were vaccinated at either 3 weeks or 10 weeks of age and their immunity assessed by challenge either 3 weeks later or at the end of the fattening period. This work showed that despite high levels of passive antibody at 3 weeks of age vaccine was still able to induce active immunization. In summary, this work provides evidence of gX deleted vaccine effectiveness in 3 areas of vaccine use which are pivotal if pseudorabies is to be controlled.

INTRODUCTION

In recent years the advent of pseudorabies virus (PRV) vaccines, which through the deletion of specific genes, give the potential to allow discrimination between vaccinated and infected animals have increased the attractiveness of vaccination/eradication policies.

The theoretical possibilities and immunological implications for such constructs are shown in Fig. 1

J. T. van Oirschot (ed.), Vaccination and Control of Aujeszky's Disease, 13–25.

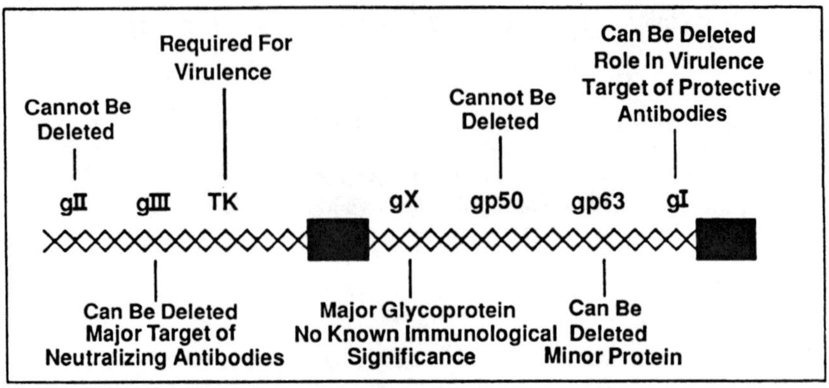

Fig. 1 Schematic representation of the PRV genome

The gX glycoprotein was first discovered by Ben-Porat and Kaplan (1970), who identified large amounts of this glycoprotein in the medium of infected cells. The gX protein is made as a cell-bound precursor which is processed presumably by proteolytic cleavage to an extracellular form (Bennett *et al.*, 1986). Our work with gX began in tests of gX as a subunit vaccine. We have produced gX in E. coli, Chinese hamster ovary cells, and in a recombinant herpes simplex virus (Post *et al.*, 1985). In each of these cases it was possible to raise high titers of anti-gX antibodies in mice. However, in no case was any neutralizing antibody detected, and very little protective effect was observed. It was then found that gX could be deleted from PRV.

Because of all of the data indicating an inability of gX to contribute to protective immunity, it seemed a logical candidate for deletion in a serologically distinguishable PRV vaccine. We have produced a vaccine strain (PRV∆TK∆gX, Tolvid®) with deletions in thymidine kinase and gX, from an otherwise wild-type PRV Aujeszky genotype (Marchioli *et al.*, 1987; Thomsen *et al.*, 1987). To detect antibodies to gX in serum of infected pigs, gX produced in E.coli was used in a simple direct ELISA test.

To further investigate the protective contribution of gX, studies were performed on the efficacy, effect on latency and use of gX deleted vaccines in the face of passive immunity plus a comparison between 2 viral constructs; one deleted at the gX region and the other at the gX and gI region.

Efficacy-Virus Shedding

The question of efficacy is complex because the perception of the value of a vaccine can change depending upon the users viewpoint and because the vaccine has to operate within the varied environments of differing pig management programs. Thus, the producer is more likely to be concerned with how well a vaccine protects against weight loss on challenge, whereas regulatory officials may be more interested in how well a vaccine prevents shedding of a challenge virus or in how well it controls latency because of the concern that vaccination should control disease spread.

The measurement of weight gain after challenge (De Leeuw and Van Oirschot, 1985a) has become an important parameter of vaccine protection against disease because it is an objective indicator of the severity of illness and directly related to economic losses. Using this measurement, and the student t-test to compare our data (Fig. 2), seronegative pigs vaccinated with PRVΔTKΔgX-1 and challenged with the Rice field strain of PRV performed considerably better than animals given a gI-negative vaccine, PR-Vac (Norden Laboratories), in that none of the PRVΔTKΔgX-1 vaccinated animals lost weight ($P = 0.001$). (Fig. 2).

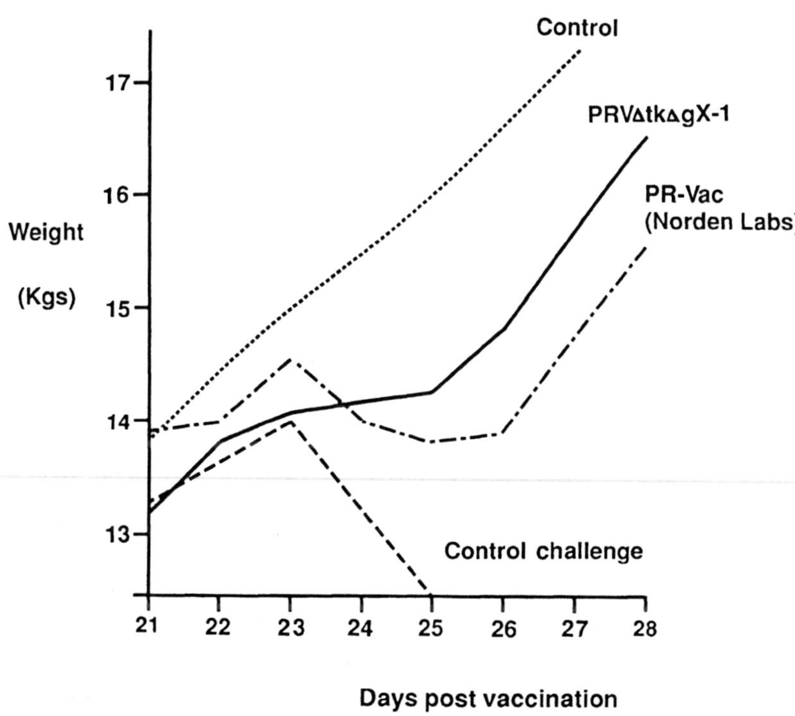

Fig. 2 Weight gain in pigs vaccinated then challenged with wild-type PRV. Four to 6-week-old piglets were IM vaccinated and challenged 3 weeks later with the Rice strain of PRV. Animals were weighed daily and each group contained 24 piglets.

Although direct side by side experiments provide the best data when comparing vaccines, it is worthy of note that other vaccine comparisons in the literature record weight loss on challenge (De Leeuw and Van Oirschot, 1985a,b), whereas this was not a feature of PRV∆TK∆gX-1 treated animals. This comparative level of protection is maintained right through the growing period with PRV∆TK∆gX-1 performing significantly better (P = 0.005) than the Bartha strain in pigs which were challenged at market weight (Fig. 3).

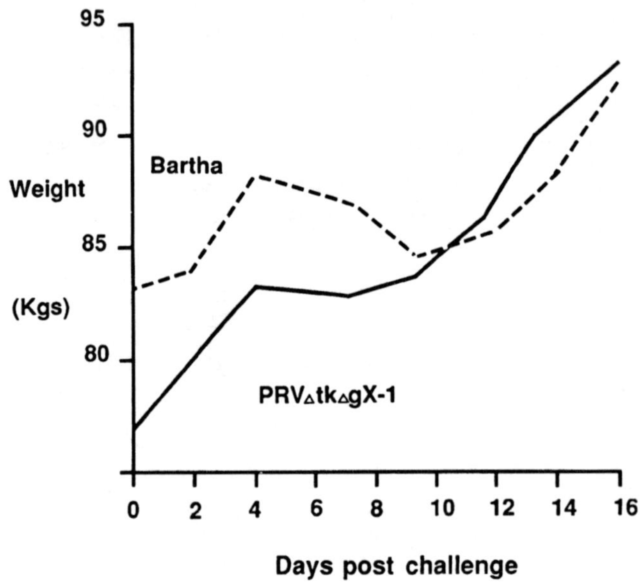

Fig. 3 Weight response of pigs vaccinated at 10-13 weeks and challenged with the Rice strain of PRV at the end of the fattening period. Each group contained 16 animals.

Virus isolation rates from challenged pigs also showed that significantly less (P = 0.001) challenge virus (Fig. 4) was found in PRV∆TK∆gX-1 vaccinates than in those given Pr-Vac (Norden Laboratories). This suggests that PRV∆TK∆gX-1 might work well under field conditions in preventing local spread of field virus within a pig house. This is a major concern in any eradication campaign as vaccines must reduce the circulation of field virus so that the overall load of potential infectious animals is reduced. In fattening house situations gI deleted vaccines do not appear to be able to do this effectively and this may be one of the reasons for those products over seeing a steady increase in the incidence of PRV over the last 15 years.

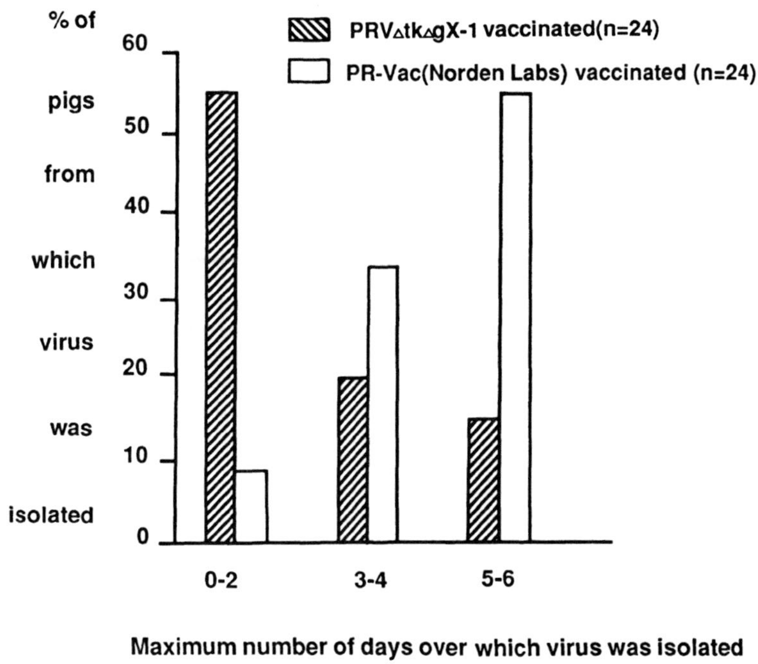

Fig. 4 Isolation of challenge virus in previously vaccinated pigs. Pigs were vaccinated and challenged 3 weeks later with the Rice strain of PRV. Challenge virus replication was monitered by oro-pharyngeal swabs, thus in over 50% of the PRVΔTKΔgX-1 vaccinated pigs, challenge virus was only isolated for 0-2 days, whereas over 50% of the Pr-Vac vaccinated animals excreted challenge virus for 5-6 days.

Latency

An ideal PRV vaccine should not only protect against disease, but should also prevent establishment of latent infection or at least reactivation of latent PRV. This is because it has been clearly shown that recrudescent PRV can infect susceptible in-contact pigs (Van Oirschot and Gielkens, 1984), and hence latently infected animals, could act as the source of virus for a new PRV outbreak. The practical importance of such animals in the epizootiology of PRV is, however, much more difficult to judge. Unlike infectious bovine rhinotracheitis viral infections of cattle and feline viral rhinotracheitis infection of cats, PRV is extremely difficult to reactivate, suggesting that latently infected pigs only rarely act as a virus source. This notion is supported by the fact that spread of virus in herds containing a few seropositive pigs is rare (Wright *et al.*, 1982). Nonetheless, seropositive latently infected pigs present a considerable problem for regulatory officials and hence any PRV vaccine which reduces recrudescence either by preventing latency or reactivation is likely to be regarded favorably.

The problem of experimentally reactivating PRV has meant that failure to isolate virus may reflect a technological problem rather than true viral absence. In a study we were uniformly successful in reactivating virus from pigs given a gp50 subunit vaccine and a subsequent challenge (Table 1). This indicates that our procedures are capable of identifying latent PRV and supports the conclusion that prior vaccination with Tolvid decreases recrudescence (Table 1).

TABLE 1 Isolation of PRV from tissues of vaccinated challenged pigs

Pig	Vaccination	Tonsil	Medulla oblongata	Lung	Bone Marrow	Trigeminal ganglia	DSC lymph node	Olfactory bulb	% Isolation rate
10	gp50	+	0	0	0	0	+	0	28
11	gp50	+	+	0	0	+	+	+	71
12	gp50	+	+	0	0	0	+	+	57
14	gp50	+	+	+	0	+	+	+	85
16	gp50	+	+	0	0	0	0	0	28
%isolation rate		100	80	20	0	40	80	60	
21	ΔTKΔgX	0	0	0	0	0	0	0	0
22	ΔTKΔgX	0	0	0	0	0	0	0	0
23	ΔTKΔgX	+	0	0	0	0	+	0	28
24	ΔTKΔgX	+	+	0	0	+	+	0	57
% isolation rate		50	25	0	0	25	50	0	

\+ = viral isolation 0 = no viral isolation

Six to 8-week-old PRV seronegative piglets were vaccinated and challenged 3 weeks later with the Rice strain of PRV. Five months later animals were treated with 1750 mg prednisolone daily for 4 days and 3 days after the final treatment animals were killed and tissues taken for virus isolation. Isolation was attempted on single cell suspensions produced by trypsin and collegenase treatment (Nesburn *et al.*, 1980) and by passing tissues through a stainless steel sieve. PK15 indicator cells were used to denote the presence of virus and all cultures were kept for at least 14 days and blind passaged at least once.

Within the context of the discussion concerning the epizootiological significance of latently infected pigs, it is pertinent to compare the performance of Tolvid vis-a-vis latency with the Bartha and Norden vaccine strains. In a study using PR-Vac (Norden Laboratories) and subsequent virus challenge, reactivated virus was found in tonsillar swabs from 5-6 pigs 90 days after challenge (Mock *et al.*, 1981). Thus, despite the probable presence of secretory antibody, virus was easily isolated from these pigs. Tissue fragments taken from these pigs were also processed by homogenization, a procedure now known to be relatively insensitive as a viral detection method (Nesburn *et al.*, 1980) and this failed to identify any further virus. This suggests that this vaccine is less efficient in preventing latency and/or reactivation and Mock *et al.* (1981) point out that their results may explain why vaccination programs have failed to eliminate the persistence and spread of virulent PRV in infected herds.

With the Bartha vaccine strain, Van Oirschot and Gielkens (1984) showed that the occurrence of latency in vaccinated pigs appeared to be reduced with a similar frequency to that of Tolvid vaccinates. However, their detection system relied upon sentinel pigs and virus isolation from tissue fragments not treated with enzymes, a procedure which is likely to be less sensitive than the method employed here (Nesburn *et al.*, 1980). It is, therefore, possible that further virus isolations would have been made if enzymatic digestion had been used.

The relative merits of a sentinel pig detection system compared to analysis of tissue fragments is a difficult issue to resolve. Spread to in-contact animals indicates epizootiological relevance, but as there is no good information on how steroid stress might compare to natural field stresses which cause reactivation, then it could be argued that the absolute detection of virus is a better indicator of the ability of vaccine to protect against latency. For instance, approximately half of our isolates were only identified after blind passage, suggesting that too small amounts of virus were present to infect susceptible in-contact pigs. These arguments support the conclusions that gX deleted vaccines will reduce the level of excretion of reactivated challenge virus and hence may be more successful in vaccine use programs for PRV control.

Vaccination and passive immunity

Breeding pigs which are kept in areas where PRV is endemic are normally vaccinated against this disease for 3 reasons. Firstly, despite the fact that adult animals often only suffer mild clinical symptoms when infected with PRV, pregnant animals can abort and thus need protection by vaccination. Secondly, vaccinated animals should be better able to control the circulation of field virus challenge and as this adds to overall herd immunity, it helps protect more susceptible piglets. Lastly, piglets will passively acquire PRV immunity from the vaccinated sow and this will protect them from disease for the early part of their life. The advantages of this protection can be offset by the fact that passive antibody has been reported to interfere with subsequent vaccination programs and hence the level of herd protection in growing swine may be significantly lower than vaccination rates would indicate. The factors involved in a vaccination program which endeavors to produce high levels of passive antibody in piglets and which can accurately forecast antibody decline in order to optimize vaccine "take", are complex and often overridden by logistical decisions of the convenience or inconvenience of administering vaccine at a particular time.

For these reasons, it was decided to evaluate the recombinantly produced live PRV vaccine PRVΔTKΔgX-1 in piglets born to immune sows by administering it at times most favored by the producer, i.e. at weaning time or when pigs enter the growing house. The usefulness of this vaccination procedure was followed by challenging piglets with field virus either 3 weeks post vaccination or at the end of the growing period.

The study showed that vaccinated gilts supply good levels of passive immunity to piglets (virus neutralizing antibody titers in piglets born to sows vaccinated before they were bred ranged from 1:128 to 1:8, mean 1:36, at 3 days of age) as evidenced by challenge at 4,7 and 10 weeks of age, and that subsequent vaccination of piglets at either 3 or 10 weeks of age provides effective immunity (Table 2) right through to the end of the fattening period.

TABLE 2 History of some piglets born to PRVΔtkΔgX-1 immune sows and then either vaccinated with PRVΔtkΔgX-1 and challenged with the Rice strain of PRV or just challenged.

Age (wks) at vaccination	Vaccinated	Challenge	Mortality
3-4	No	Yes	6/15*
3-4	Yes	Yes	0/21
10-13	No	Yes	11/14
10-13	Yes	Yes	0/20

* PRV seronegative 3-4 week old piglets experience over 90% mortality when challenged with the Rice strain.

It is of interest to note, however, that performance analysis at the end of the growing period shows an advantage to 10-week-old vaccination, as although both groups performed well, the 3-week-old vaccinates did lose significantly ($p = 0.001$)

more weight, 5.7 kilos to 2.2 kilos and experienced a significantly ($p = 0.001$) longer period of growth arrest, 8.5 days to 3.6 days. This difference may reflect either a diminished ability of the vaccine to engender a full immune response in the face of high levels of passive immunity, although it is obviously sufficient to give extremely good protection against growth arrest and mortality 3 weeks later, or the 7 week time difference between the 2 vaccinations means that at the end of the fattening period, the immunity stimulated at 3 weeks would have declined somewhat more than that stimulated at 10 weeks and hence, the pigs showed a different response when challenged. The significance of this for the producer depends on the epidemiological pattern of PRV associated with his particular production unit. Often, for reasons which have not been fully explained, disease on a particular farm is associated more with 1 age group of pigs than another. Hence, if the producer is having problems mainly in the nursery house (4 to 10-week-old pigs) it may be advisable to vaccinate weaned pigs at 3 to 4 weeks of age. If, on the other hand, problems are associated with pigs nearing the end of the growth period, then vaccination at 10 weeks would give optimum protection.

Although the literature contains many reports which indicate that passive immunity severely interferes with vaccination, it is difficult to make direct comparisons between how well individual PRV vaccines perform unless they are compared in exactly similar trials. It is interesting to note, however, that in 1 report (Vannier, 1985) piglets born to immune sows and vaccinated between 8 and 10 weeks of age all lost more weight on challenge at the end of the growth period than Tolvid 3-week-old vaccinates. Another report shows seroconversion rates as low as 20% in piglets vaccinated at 15 weeks of age with seroconversion rates often below 50% even when piglets were vaccinated twice (Pensaert and Maes, 1984). Similarly, Wright *et al.* (1984) have shown that titers only increased after vaccination in piglets of at least 12 weeks of age. This suggests that Tolvid may be markedly superior in overcoming passive immunity to provide protection right through to the end of the growth phase.

Protective contribution of gX and gI

Most conventional PRV vaccines already have a deletion of gI as this gene is readily lost upon viral passage (Mettenleiter *et al.*,1987). The fact that these vaccines have been used for many years and that their field characteristics are well understood argues for their continued use in any eradication program. However, it is now known that gI contributes not only to virulence (Berns *et al.*, 1985), (in a virus where gI represents the major gene deletion) but that pigs may make an immune response to this protein which contributes toward protection against subsequent wild virus challenge. Evidence for this comes from the fact that monoclonal antibodies which react with gI will, when administered to mice, protect them against wild-type virus. It could be argued, however, that as pigs respond to many other proteins coded for by the PRV that the contribution made by gI is so small that its deletion is not going to affect vaccine efficacy. When a gX deleted virus produced by recombinant DNA technology from a fully virulent parent has been compared in efficacy experiments with a number of conventionally produced gI deleted vaccines (see efficacy section), the gX deleted vaccine has always shown far superior efficacy. These results strongly suggest that any eradication program based on gI deleted vaccines will not be as effective as using a gX deleted vaccine because of the importance of gI in the immune response. However, the conventionally produced gI vaccines are known to have further modifications of their genome (Ben-Porat *et al.*, 1986) as a result of tissue culture passage and hence, their inferior performance could in part be due to these modifications rather than the loss of gI. Direct evidence for this conclusion can only be drawn from a comparison of 2 vaccines which have an identical make-up apart from being either gXgI negative or solely gX negative.

Thus, 62 4 to 6-week-old PRV free piglets were vaccinated with the vaccine PRVΔTKΔgX. A further 79 piglets were similarly vaccinated with PRVΔTKΔgX in which a further deletion of gI had been made giving a virus designated PRVΔTKΔgXΔgI. After 3 weeks, animals were challenged intranasally with the Rice strain of PRV and piglets were monitered for clinical signs. Pigs given the gI deleted vaccine showed significantly greater growth arrest ($P=0.026$), lost significantly more weight ($P=0.006$) and for a longer period of time ($P=0.015$) than those given the vaccine containing gI. Similarly, gI deleted vaccinates shed more challenge virus ($P=0.001$) and showed a greater pyrexic response on challenge ($P=0.006$).

These results show that the absence of the gI gene results in a vaccine virus which is significantly inferior to a virus which contains that gene. This result is of interest at 2 levels. Firstly, it gives significant information in the host animal species on the relative importance of this gene in producing an immune response and secondly, it reflects upon the use of different vaccine/diagnostic packages for the possible eradication of PRV. It is known that gI is required for the expression of virulence in some animal systems and also that gI monoclonal antibodies protect mice against lethal PRV challenge. This glycoprotein thus has a dual role. The gX glycoprotein, on the other hand, has no assigned biological role (Marchioli *et al.*, 1987) and despite its abundance production does not appear to induce a protective immune response. From a theoretical standpoint therefore, gX deletions might not be expected to have an effect on immunity, whereas gI deletions would. Our results support this hypothesis and indicate that as well as gIII, gI must now be considered as a major target for a protective response (Ben-Porat *et al.*,1986). It has also been shown that gI expression affects replication of the virus in some model systems (Lomniczi *et al.*, 1984). If this is also true in the pig, then this could also contribute to the poor performance of gI deleted vaccines.

There is also the possibility that the dual deletion of gX and gI could have synergistically affected the immunogenicity of that virus construct and hence the observed effect was not solely due to the absence of gI. Although synergistic effects of glycoprotein deletions have been reported (Schreurs *et al.*, 1988), since gX is a non-structural protein this seems unlikely in this case. In interpreting deletion experiments, it is important to keep in mind that deletion of one gene, especially a gene encoding a major structural protein, could have an effect on the overall configuration of the virus and so change the immunogenic dominance of one protein compared to another. Although this caveat must be kept in mind in interpretation of experiments, these methodologies provide the best tool available for investigating the immunological role of individual proteins.

CONCLUSIONS

In any PRV eradication program in which vaccines are going to be used, it would be sensible to use a product which gave the maximum protection from wild virus challenge. From the producers point of view, this means less weight loss on virulent challenge and from the regulatory standpoint better control of the replication of challenge virus and of the possibility of reactivation. This data supports the claim that gX deleted vaccines are superior to gI deleted products on both those counts.

The control of PRV is a difficult task and any program using vaccines as its base should use the best available product. This data and the fact that the past 12 years of gI deleted vaccine use has seen a steady increase in the incidence of PRV, makes gX deleted vaccines a compelling choice for eradication program use.

REFERENCES

Bennett, L.M., Timmins, J.G., Thomsen, D.R. and Post, L.E. 1986. The processing of pseudorabies virus glycoprotein gX in infected cells and in an uninfected cell line. Virol., **155,** 707-715.

Ben-Porat, T. and Kaplan, A.S. 1970. Synthesis of proteins in cells infected with herpes virus. Virol., **41,** 265-273.

Ben-Porat, T., DeMarchi, J.M., Lomniczi, B. and Kaplan, A.S. 1986. Role of glycoproteins of pseudorabies virus in eliciting neutralizing antibodies. Virol., **154**, 325-334.

Berns, A., Van den Ouweland, A., Quint, W., Van Oirschot, J.T. and Gielkens, A.L.J. 1985. Presence of markers for virulence in the unique short region or repeat region or both of pseudorabies hybrid viruses. J. Virol., **53,** 89-93.

De Leeuw, P.W. and Van Oirschot, J.T. 1985a. Vaccines against Aujeszky's disease: Evaluation of their efficacy under standardized laboratory conditions. Vet. Quarterly, **7,** 191-197.

De Leeuw, P.W. and Van Oirschot, J.T. 1985b. Intranasal vaccination of pigs with Aujeszky's disease: Comparison with inactivated vaccines in pigs with low maternal antibody titers. Res. Vet. Sci., **39,** 34-38.

Lomniczi, B., Watanabe, S., Ben-Porat, T. and Kaplan, A.S. 1984. Genetic basis of the neurovirulence of pseudorabies virus. J. Virol., **52,** 198-205.

Marchioli, C.C., Yancey, Jr., R.J., Wardley, R.C., Thomsen, D.R. and Post, L.E. 1987. A vaccine strain of pseudorabies virus with deletions in the thymidine kinase and glycoprotein X genes. Am. J. Vet. Res., **48,** 1577-1583.

Mettenleiter, T.C., Schreurs, C., Thiel, H.J. and Rziha, H.J. 1987. Variability of pseudorabies virus glycoprotein I expression. Virol., **158,** 141-146.

Mock, R.E., Crandell, R.A. and Mesfin, G.M. 1981. Induced latency in pseudorabies vaccinated pigs. Can. J. Comp. Med., **45,** 56-59.

Nesburn, A.B., Dunkel, E.C. and Trousdale, M.D. 1980. Enhanced herpes simplex virus recovery from neuronal tissues of latently infected rabbits. Proc. Soc. Exp. Biol. Med., **163,** 398-401.

Pensaert, M.B. and Maes, L. 1984. Parenteral and intranasal vaccination of fattening pigs against Aujeszky's disease. ZbL. Vet. Med. B., **31,** 682-689.

Post, L.E., Marchioli, C.C., Timmins, J.G., Thomsen, D.R. and Yancey, Jr., R.J. 1985. Recombinant HSV expressing pseudorabies virus glycoprotein genes. 10th International herpes virus workshop, Ann Arbor, MI. p. 201.

Schreurs, C., Mettenleiter, T.C., Zuckerman, F., Sugg, N. and Ben-Porat, T. 1988. Glycoprotein gIII of pseudorabies virus is multifunctional. J. Virol., **62,** 2251-2257.

Thomsen, D.R., Marchioli, C.C., Yancey, Jr., R.J. and Post, L.E. 1987. Replication and virulence of pseudorabies virus mutants lacking glycoprotein gX. J. Virol., **61,** 229-232.

Vannier, P. 1985. Experimental infection of fattening pigs with pseudorabies virus: Efficacy of attenuated live - and inactivated virus vaccines in pigs with or without passive immunity. Am. J. Vet. Res., **46,** 1498-1502.

Van Oirschot, J.T. and Gielkens, A.L.J. 1984. Intranasal vaccination of pigs against pseudorabies: Absence of vaccinal virus latency and failure to prevent latency of virulent virus. Am. J. Vet. Res., **45,** 2099-2103.

Wright, J.C., Thawley, D.G. and Solorzano, R.F. 1982. Field evaluation of test- and -removal and vaccination as control measures for pseudorabies in Missouri swine. Can. J. Comp. Med., **46,** 420-425.

Wright, J.C., Thawley, D.G. and Solorzano, R.F. 1984. Immune response of sows and their offspring to pseudorabies virus: Serum neutralisation response to vaccination and field virus challenge. Can. J. Comp. Med., **48,** 184-191.

VACCINE EFFICACY AND INNOCUITY OF STRAIN 783 OF AUJESZKY'S DISEASE VIRUS

A.L.J. Gielkens, R.J.M. Moormann*, J.T. van Oirschot*, A.J.M. Berns***

* Central Veterinary Institute, Department of Virology, Houtribweg 39, 8221 RA Lelystad, The Netherlands
** Netherlands Cancer Institute, Section of Molecular Genetics, Plesmanlaan 121, 1066 CX Amsterdam, The Netherlands

ABSTRACT

A glycoprotein I (gI) and thymidine kinase (TK) deletion mutant of the Aujeszky's disease virus (ADV) strain NIA-3 was constructed. The mutant, designated ADV 783, was examined for vaccine efficacy and innocuity.

A single intramuscular vaccination of seronegative pigs with 10^5 plaque-forming units (PFU) of ADV strain 783 conferred almost complete protection against challenge with 10^5 PFU of virulent ADV, 12 weeks after vaccination. Maternally immune pigs vaccinated twice intramuscularly and challenged 12 weeks after the first vaccination showed mild signs of disease and loss of appetite for 3 to 4 days.

No adverse reactions were observed after intranasal and intramuscular inoculation of piglets, sheep, and calves with 10^7 PFU of ADV 783. After intranasal and intramuscular inoculation of pregnant sows with 10^7 PFU of ADV 783, no adverse reactions were seen during gestation and no evidence was found for transmission of virus across the placenta. Furthermore, no indications were found that ADV 783 established latent infections in piglets.

INTRODUCTION

The construction of a deletion mutant of the NIA-3 strain of Aujeszky's disease (AD) virus (ADV) has been described (Quint *et al.*, 1987). The mutant virus, designated 2.4N3A, contains deletions of 2055 base pairs (bp) in the unique short region of the genome and of about 100 bp at the Hind III sites in both inverted repeats. The region within the unique short region that is deleted from the 2.4N3A genome, spans the gene coding for the structural glycoprotein I (gI) and part of the coding sequences of the 11K protein (Berns *et al.*, unpublished data).

Although the 2.4N3A strain of ADV is strongly reduced in virulence, it still caused disease in 4-day-old ADV-seronegative piglets. Further attenuation of ADV 2.4N3A was established by introducing a small deletion into the 3'-coding region of the thymidine kinase (TK) gene (Moormann *et al.*, in preparation). A mutant virus

J. T. van Oirschot (ed.), Vaccination and Control of Aujeszky's Disease, 27–35.

containing a 19 bp deletion within the TK gene was selected. This gI^-/TK^- mutant, designated ADV 783, was examined for vaccine efficacy and innocuity. In this paper we report only the most important findings. Details on the construction and the vaccine properties of ADV 783 will be reported elsewhere.

MATERIALS AND METHODS

Experimental animals

Seronegative pigs were from the "minimal disease" Dutch landrace herd of the Central Veterinary Institute, which is free of AD. Maternally immune pigs and seronegative sows, sheep and calves were from privately owned herds. The maternally immune pigs had been born to sows repeatedly vaccinated with the Bartha vaccine virus and were negative for antibodies against gI.

Sampling procedures, virus titrations and neutralization tests

Collection of blood and oropharyngeal fluid (OPF) samples, virus titrations and neutralization tests were done as described previously (De Leeuw *et al.*, 1982).

RESULTS

Vaccine efficacy of ADV 783 in seronegative pigs

Seronegative pigs were vaccinated intramuscularly (IM) with 10^5 PFU of the ADV strains 2.4N3A or 783 or with a vaccine based on the Bartha strain (Ingelvac®, Boehringer Ingelheim, USA) at the age of 10 weeks. On postvaccination day 1, a sentinel pig was added to each group. A 4th group served as unvaccinated controls.

After vaccination, none of the pigs in the 4 experimental groups showed signs of illness or a reduced growth rate. The average body temperatures of the pigs given ADV 783 and Bartha remained below 40°C. The 2.4N3A inoculated pigs, however, had an average body temperature above 40°C for 2 days. All vaccinated pigs developed virus-neutralizing (VN) antibodies to ADV. The mean VN titer of the 2.4N3A inoculated group was considerably higher than that of the other groups (Table 1). After vaccination, no virus excretion was found and all sentinel pigs remained seronegative.

Twelve weeks after vaccination, pigs were challenged by intranasal (IN) instillation of 10^5 PFU of virulent NIA-3 virus (De Leeuw *et al.*, 1982). Control pigs developed signs of illness characteristic for AD, but none of the pigs died. The 2.4N3A and 783 vaccinates (except 4 of 8 pigs that showed very mild signs of disease for 1 to 2 days) did not have clinical signs of AD and the groups' average body temperatures remained below 40°C. The mean growth curves of both groups were unaffected by the challenge (Fig. 1). Bartha vaccinated pigs showed a short period of fever and a mean growth arrest period of 7 days (Table 1).

TABLE 1 Vaccine efficacy of ADV 783 in seronegative pigs

Vaccine	Mean VN-titer[a] PCD[c] 0	14	No. dead/ No. tested	Mean days of growth arrest	fever[b]	virus shedding
783	1.6	2.4	0/8	0	0	0
2.4N3A	2.3	2.3	0/8	0	0	0
Bartha	1.6	3.5	0/8	7	2	2
Controls	—	2.5	0/8	14	7	7

[a] VN: virus neutralization ($\log_{10}$)
[b] Fever: body temperature above 40°C
[c] Postchallenge day

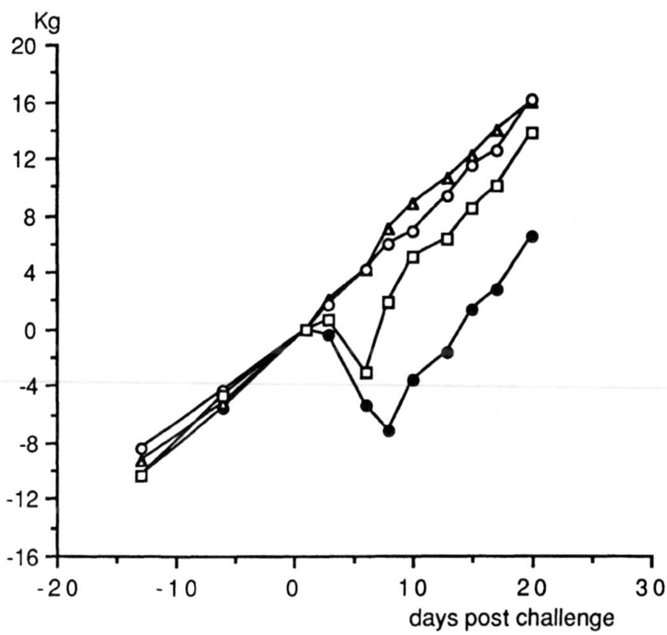

Fig. 1 Mean weight curves (n = 8) before and after challenge exposure of seronegative pigs that were given ADV strain 2.4N3A (Δ-Δ), 783 (o-o), or Bartha (□–□). Unvaccinated controls of the same age (●-●).

Shedding of the challenge virus was prevented in the pigs vaccinated with ADV strains 2.4N3A and 783. In contrast, 1 of 4 Bartha vaccinated pigs shed virus for 2 days and control pigs for 7 days.

After challenge, all control pigs seroconverted and all Bartha vaccinated pigs showed a marked secondary antibody response. On the other hand, only 4 of 8 pigs vaccinated with 783 and none of the 2.4N3A vaccinates had a secondary antibody response after challenge.

Vaccine efficacy of ADV 783 in maternally immune pigs

Ten-week-old pigs with high levels of maternal antibody (mean VN-titer 1.65) were IM vaccinated with 10^5 PFU of the ADV strains 783 or Bartha (CDI strain, De Leeuw *et al.*, 1982). Four weeks later, pigs were revaccinated in the same manner. One group of maternally immune pigs served as unvaccinated control.

The groups were challenged 12 weeks after the first vaccination and monitored for 3 weeks for clinical signs, body temperatures, growth rate, and virus shedding. Control pigs developed signs of disease for 9-16 days, but none of the pigs died. Pigs vaccinated with ADV 783 had mild signs of disease as dullness, fever, and loss of appetite lasting for an average of 4 days (Table 2). Clinical signs in the Bartha vaccinates were more severe and lasted longer. This observation was confirmed by the weight curves (Fig. 2). The control pigs needed 17 days to regain the group's mean weight they had at day 1 after challenge, the 783 vaccinates needed 6 days and the Bartha vaccinates 9 days.

TABLE 2 Vaccine efficacy of ADV 783 in maternally immune pigs

Vaccine	Mean VN-titer[a] PCD[c]		No. dead/ No. tested	Mean days of		
	0	14		growth arrest	fever[b]	virus shedding
783	1.6	3.5	0/8	6	3	5
Bartha	1.2	3.5	0/8	9	4	5
Controls	0.2	2.4	0/8	17	7	$\geq$10

[a] VN: virus neutralization ($\log_{10}$)
[b] Fever: body temperature above 40°C
[c] Postchallenge day

Both vaccinated groups showed a reduced period of virus shedding compared to the controls. However, the mean virus titers in OPF samples of the 783 vaccinated pigs were 10-100 fold lower than in those of the Bartha vaccinates (Fig. 3).

After challenge, the VN-antibody titers of pigs in both vaccinated groups rose rapidly.

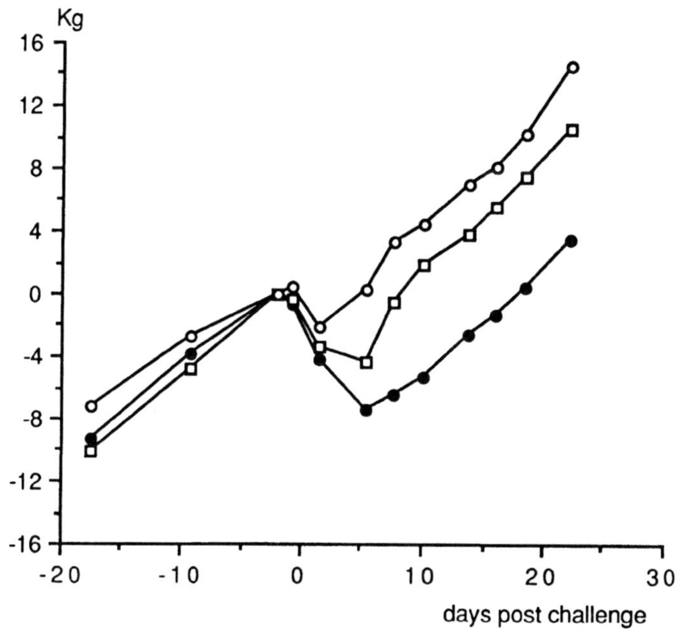

Fig. 2 Mean weight curves (n = 7-8) before and after challenge exposure. Maternally immune pigs given vaccine strain ADV 783 (o-o), or Bartha (□–□). Unvaccinated controls of the same age (●-●).

Innocuity of ADV 783 for piglets, sheep and calves

To examine innocuity of ADV 783, seronegative piglets, sheep and calves were exposed to a high virus dose. Briefly, each of 4 pigs, 4 days of age, were inoculated both IN and IM with $10^{6.7}$ PFU of virus. Two groups of 4 sheep, 6-7 months old, received 10^7 PFU of virus by the IN or IM route. The innocuity test in 4-week-old specific-pathogen-free calves was performed in the same manner as that in sheep.

During the observation period, postvaccination days 0-21, no clinical signs suggestive of AD were observed in any of the inoculated animals. None of the groups of animals showed marked rises in average body temperatures. Only the IN inoculated sheep had body temperatures just above 40°C at day 2 after inoculation. All animals, except the IN inoculated calves, developed VN antibodies to ADV.

No reactivation of ADV 783

In order to establish whether ADV 783 induces a latent infection, 4-day-old seronegative pigs, were inoculated both IN and IM with $10^{6.7}$ PFU of virus. To reactivate putative latent ADV, pigs were subjected to immunosuppressive treatment (Van Oirschot and Gielkens, 1984). Pigs were treated for 4 consecutive days starting on day 46 after inoculation. At the start of the treatment, 2 ADV seronegative pigs were introduced into the group to act as sentinels. Immunosuppressed and sentinel pigs were monitored daily for clinical signs and body temperatures. In addition, OPF samples were collected daily for 3 weeks and blood samples were taken weekly. On day 25 after the start of the treatment, the pigs were sacrificed and pieces of brain, mandibular lymph nodes, tonsil, and lung were taken and assayed for infectious virus. Explant cultures of trigeminal ganglia were examined as described previously (Van Oirschot and Gielkens, 1984).

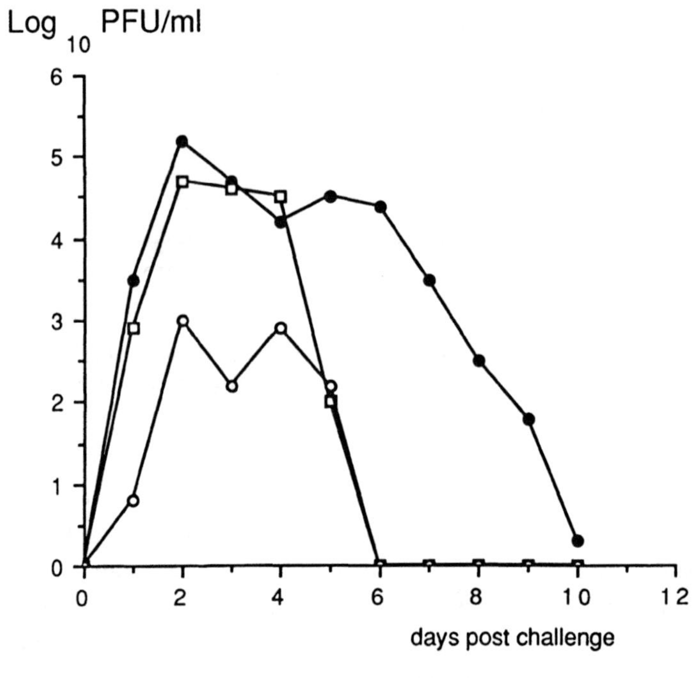

Fig. 3 Mean virus excretion curves after challenge exposure. In each group, 4 pigs were sampled. Maternally immune pigs given vaccine strain ADV 783 (o-o), or Bartha (□—□). Unvaccinated controls of the same age (●-●).

After corticosteroid treatment, no clinical signs of AD were observed. All OPF samples collected, were negative for infectious ADV. Furthermore, no ADV was recovered from tissue specimens obtained postmortem from the inoculated pigs. None of the explant cultures of trigeminal ganglia from these pigs produced virus. Vaccinated and immunosuppressed pigs did not show a secondary antibody response and sentinel pigs remained seronegative throughout the observation period.

No transmission of ADV 783 across the placenta

To examine whether ADV 783 is capable to cross the placenta, seronegative pregnant sows were inoculated both IN and IM with 10^7 PFU of virus. Four sows of group A received virus at day 85 of gestation and 5 sows of group B at day 34 or 35 of gestation. At the end of gestation, piglets born to the vaccinated sows of group A were sacrificed. Specimens of brain, mandibular lymph nodes, tonsil, lung, liver, and spleen were collected from all piglets and assayed for virus. Group B sows were sacrificed at day 70 of gestation. At this time, tissue specimens were collected from all fetuses and subjected to virus isolation. Blood samples were taken from all sows before inoculation and at the end of the experiment, and from the baby pigs immediately after birth.

After inoculation, none of the sows developed clinical signs of AD. Furthermore, the vaccine virus did not cause adverse reactions during pregnancy. At necropsy, no infectious ADV was recovered from tissue specimens collected from both piglets and fetuses. All vaccinated sows developed VN antibodies to ADV. None of the piglets born to the vaccinated sows had antibodies in precolostral sera.

No reversion to virulence of ADV 783

To examine whether avirulence is a stably acquired property of ADV 783, the virus was passaged in 3 to 5-day-old piglets. Two seronegative piglets were each inoculated both IN and IM with 10^7 PFU of ADV 783. Four days later, the pigs were sacrificed and tissue specimens were made from brain, lymph nodes, lung, tonsil, and liver.

Virus-positive organ suspensions were pooled and administered into 2 piglets in the same manner as described for the first passage. This operation was repeated until the virus disappeared.

At the 3rd passage, no infectious ADV was recovered. Therefore, a second series of passages was carried out. Again the virus disappeared, but this time at the 4th passage.

DISCUSSION

Genetic engineering procedures were employed to attenuate the wild-type ADV strain NIA-3 by deletion mutation. One deletion spans the coding regions of the viral glycoprotein gI and part of the viral 11K protein. The second deletion inactivates the TK gene, which is required for infection of neural tissues.

Studies of Quint *et al.* (1987) showed that inactivation of gI has a marked effect on the virulence of ADV in 10-week-old pigs. However, gI^- deletion mutants are still moderately virulent in 3-week-old pigs (Mettenleiter *et al.*, 1987) and in pigs younger than 1 week of age (Van Oirschot, unpublished results). Further attenuation of the gI^- deletion mutant 2.4N3A was established by introducing a deletion into the TK gene (Moormann *et al.*, in preparation). A TK^- derivative of 2.4N3A, designated as ADV 783, with a 19 bp deletion from within the TK coding sequences, was examined for vaccine efficacy and innocuity.

The efficacy evaluation demonstrated that a single IM vaccination of seronegative pigs with 10^5 PFU of ADV 783, was highly effective in preventing clinical signs, virus shedding, and growth arrest after challenge exposure 12 weeks after vaccination. In the same experiment, a vaccine based on the Bartha strain induced a moderate protection, whereas ADV strain 2.4N3A conferred complete protection. The better protective immunity of the 2.4N3A vaccinates is most likely due to the higher *in vivo* replication efficiency of this TK^+ deletion mutant compared with that of the TK^- derivative. As expected, the efficacy of ADV 783 decreased when tested in pigs with high levels of maternally derived antibodies. After challenge, mild signs of disease were recorded as dullness, fever, and reduced food intake. Nevertheless, vaccination markedly shortened the period of growth arrest and virus shedding. Notably, the amount of challenge virus shed was 10-100 fold lower in ADV 783 vaccinated pigs than in Bartha vaccinated pigs.

The innocuity evaluation of ADV 783 permits the conclusion that the virus can safely be administered to seronegative pigs of all ages and to pregnant sows. The absence of any adverse reaction in sheep and calves vaccinated both IM and IN with 10^7 PFU of virus, confirms the high degree of attenuation of ADV 783.

Other criteria that live ADV vaccines have to fulfil, are absence of latency induction and genetic stability following passage in pigs. Reactivation of ADV 783 in pigs could not be demonstrated. This finding indicates that the capacity of ADV 783 to induce a latent state is impeded. Because the avirulence of ADV 783 was affected by deletion of genes, it is highly unlikely that reversion to virulence occurs following passage in pigs. This hypothesis is corroborated by the disappearance of the virus following 3 or 4 passages in piglets.

In conclusion, the gI^-/TK^- deletion mutant ADV 783 was shown to be a safe and highly effective vaccine in pigs. Because the virus does not induce antibodies to gI, vaccinated pigs can be distinguished from those infected with wild-type virus.

Recent data (Van Oirschot and De Waal, 1987; Van Oirschot and Wijsmuller, 1988) provide evidence that a program of continuing vaccination with gI^- vaccines followed by testing for antibodies to gI and culling of gI-seropositive pigs, can be successfully applied in control and eradication of ADV.

ACKNOWLEDGEMENTS

We thank F. Daus, J. Briaire, A.P. de Rover, and M. van der Palen for skilful technical assistance. This investigation was supported by the Netherlands Technology Foundation, Duphar BV, Intervet International BV, and Gist-Brocades NV.

REFERENCES

De Leeuw, P.W., Wijsmuller, J.M., Zantinga, J.W. and Tielen, M.J.M. 1982. Intranasal vaccination of pigs against Aujeszky's disease. 1. Comparison of intranasal or parenteral vaccination with an attenuated vaccine in 12-week-old pigs from immunized dams. Vet. Quarterly **4,** 49-56.

Mettenleiter, T.C., Zsak, L., Kaplan, A.S., Ben-Porat, T. and Lomniczi, B. 1987. Role of a structural glycoprotein of pseudorabies in virus virulence. J. Virol., **61,** 4030-4032.

Quint, W., Gielkens, A.L.J., Van Oirschot, J.T., Berns, A. and Cuypers, T. 1987. Construction and characterization of deletion mutants of pseudorabies virus: a new generation of 'live' vaccines. J. Gen. Virol., **68,** 523-534.

Van Oirschot, J.T. and Gielkens, A.L.J. 1984. In vivo and in vitro reactivation of latent pseudorabies virus in pigs born to vaccinated sows. Am. J. Vet. Res., **45,** 567-571.

Van Oirschot, J.T. and De Waal, C.A.H. 1987. An ELISA to distinguish between Aujeszky's disease vaccinated and infected pigs. Vet. Rec., **121,** 305-306.

Van Oirschot, J.T. and Wijsmuller, J.M. 1988. Monitoring of a vaccinated pig breeding herd for antibody to glycoprotein I of Aujeszky's disease virus. Proc. 10th IPVS Congress, Rio de Janeiro. p. 172.

EXPERIENCES WITH A gI^-/TK^- MODIFIED LIVE PSEUDORABIES VIRUS VACCINE: STRAIN BEGONIA

N. Visser, D. Lütticken

Intervet International B.V., Akzo Pharma Division,
P.O. Box 31, 5830 AA Boxmeer, The Netherlands

ABSTRACT

Recent progress in molecular biology provided the opportunity to design a live pseudorabies virus vaccine, that pairs a high immunogenicity with avirulence. This vaccine also enables us to differentiate, by a serological assay, between infected or vaccinated pigs. This report highlights the results on efficacy and safety of the (gI^-/TK^-) pseudorabies virus vaccine strain Begonia. The strain Begonia has been shown to be safe for pigs of all ages (including pregnant sows), for other farm animals and for pet animals. Its efficacy was tested under various conditions and especially a standardized challenge model showed that the strain completely protected against excretion of challenge virus and a noticeable growth retardation. In laboratory experiments and field experiences where over 1.5 million doses of this vaccine were used no adverse reactions were noticed.

INTRODUCTION

Recent progress in DNA-recombinant techniques to modify viruses has provided the opportunity to more precisely define the characteristics of a vaccine virus. A pseudorabies virus (PRV) vaccine was developed, in which we aimed for an immunogenicity comparable to that of field strains, but at the same time it should be safe for pigs of all ages as well as for other farm and pet animals. To this end Quint *et al.* (1987) constructed a derivative of the field isolate NIA-3, which lacks the gene for glycoprotein I (gI).

The absence of gI on the surface of the virion has 2 consequences; firstly, a reduction of virulence and secondly, the possibility, by detecting antibodies to gI, to distinguish between vaccinated or infected pigs. From this deletion mutant, called 2.4N3A, a thymidine kinase (TK) defective mutant was selected via bromo-deoxyuridine screening. The resulting vaccine strain Begonia is the subject of this report, in which we have focussed on safety and immunity in laboratory tests and general aspects of large scale applications in the field.

J. T. van Oirschot (ed.), Vaccination and Control of Aujeszky's Disease, 37–44.

RESULTS AND DISCUSSION

Safety

In a series of experiments, summarized in Table 1, we have shown that in very young, susceptible and healthy piglets, from 2 days of age no adverse effects are induced by application of strain Begonia in high doses, up to 10^8 $TCID_{50}$, intranasally (IN) and intramuscularly (IM) at the same time.

TABLE 1 Safety of PRV strain Begonia in seronegative pigs

Pigs		Administration		Mortality-Symptoms of/total number	Remarks
Age	Status	Route	Dose ($TCID_{50}$)		
< 1 week		IM + IN*	10^6-10^8	0/45	Seroconversion
4-10 weeks		IM + IN	10^6	0/51	Seroconversion
sows	D40/80 of pregnancy	IM + IN	10^6	0/10	Seroconversion of sows. Fetuses no abnormalities and seronegative

*IM = intramuscularly
IN = intranasally

Pregnant sows vaccinated at day 40 or day 80 of gestation showed no abnormal reaction. Examination of the litters 3 weeks later revealed seronegative, virus-free healthy fetuses. At that time the sows had seroconverted to an average virus neutralization (VN) antibody titer of 32. Local and systemic reactions, like depression, were absent, and also temperatures were not different from unvaccinated controls.

Survival of 2-day-old piglets after intracerebral inoculation with $10^{5.3}$ $TCID_{50}$ of PRV is also considered a measure of safety for PRV vaccines. As shown in Table 2, the vaccine was completely safe by this criterion: the piglet intracerebral LD_{50} of strain Begonia was $10^{5.6}$.

The safety in other farm and pet animals was studied and is presented in Tables 3 and 4. High doses (10^6 $TCID_{50}$/animal) did not affect calves and sheep. Surprisingly, no significant seroconversion was observed in the VN test after 1 inoculation. On the other hand, cats and dogs seroconverted after IM injection of the same dose. There were no adverse reactions in the cats, but 2 of the 5 dogs developed clinical Aujeszky's disease. The oral administration of the vaccine strain to dogs was completely safe (Table 4). This route is of relevance if contaminated pigmeat is consumed by dogs.

TABLE 2 Intracerebral inoculation of 2-day-old piglets with 0.1 ml of serial dilutions of Begonia strain vaccine virus, batch 77126. Piglet ICLD50: calculated according to Spearman-Kärber.

Dose ($log_{10}TCID_{50}$)	Deaths/Total
6.3	5/6
5.3	0/4
4.3	0/4
diluent	0/4

TABLE 3 Safety of PRV strain Begonia in farm animals

Species	Administration		Mortality-Symptoms of/ total number	Remarks
	Route	Dose ($TCID_{50}$)		
Cattle	IM + IN	10^6	0/4	6 weeks of age, no significant seroconversion
Sheep	IM	10^6	0/5	Over 1 year of age No significant seroconversion

TABLE 4 Safety of PRV strain Begonia in pets

Species	Administration		Mortality-Symptoms of/ total number	Remarks
	Route	Dose ($TCID_{50}$)		
Dogs	IM	10^6	2/5	Seroconversion in survivors
Dogs	oral	10^6	0/6	No seroconversion
Cats	IM	10^6	0/6	All seroconverted

As expected for a gI^-/TK^- vaccine strain, Begonia was completely innocuous for day-old chickens at 10^5 $TCID_{50}$/dose, and for mice even 10^8 $TCID_{50}$/dose did not reveal any virulence (Table 5).

Rabbits seemed to be more susceptible for this highly attenuated pseudorabies strain since 5 out of 8 animals died. Nevertheless, pathogenicity was strongly reduced, if one compares the mean-time-to-death (MTD) for Begonia (144 hours) with the MTD for field isolates (58 hours) (Platt *et al.*, 1979).

TABLE 5 Safety of PRV strain Begonia in laboratory animals

Species	Administration		Mortality-Symptoms of/ total number	Remarks
	Route	Dose ($TCID_{50}$)		
Mice	IM/SC*	10^6-10^8	0/>500	Swiss, C57BL/10
Chicken	IC*	10^5	0/39	1 day of age
Rabbits	IM	10^6	5/8	Reduced pathogenicity MTD* = 144 h

* MTD = mean-time-to-death; *SC = subcutaneously; *IC = intracerebrally.

Latency

Latency is a typical characteristic of PRV. Whether the lack of this characteristic is an advantage for a vaccine strain, is still a matter of dispute.

We examined the possible establishment of latency of the Begonia virus in 2 different experiments, one using piglets vaccinated at 5 days of age and another in which 4-week-old piglets were inoculated. Three months after vaccination the pigs were treated with prednisolone (15 mg/kg body weight) for 4 consecutive days. Three weeks after the treatment organ tissues were examined for reactivated virus by trying to reisolate virus from these tissues. In one experiment brain tissues were also examined via hybridization with viral probes (H.J. Rziha, Tübingen). The results of the latency studies are summarized in Table 6.

In none of the animals any sign of reactivated virus was found, nor could the presence of viral genomes be detected via hybridization.

TABLE 6 Two experiments were performed with piglets of different ages to determine the presence of latent virus in vaccinated piglets by reactivation with prednisolone treatment.

	Exp.1	Exp.2
Age at vaccination	4 weeks	5 days
Number of animals	7	5
Dose	10^5	10^6
Prednisolone treatment	15 mg/kg	15 mg/kg
Time after vaccination	3.5 months	3.0 months
Number of sentinels	2	4
Reactivated virus		
in nasal swabs	all negative	all negative
in homogenates[1]	all negative	all negative
in cocultivations[2]	not done	all negative
Hybridization[3]	not done	all negative
Sentinels after 3 weeks	seronegative	seronegative

[1]. brain, lung, tonsils, lymph nodes
[2]. tonsils, ganglia trigeminale
[3]. brain, ganglia trigeminale, bulbus, medulla.

Spread of virus

In various experiments under controlled conditions, groups of 60 pigs, vaccinated up to 7 weeks of age, were kept in direct contact with 30 controls. Only 1 case of virus transmission between pigs was observed, in which 4 IN + IM inoculated piglets (less than 1 week old) were left with the sow, together with 2 control pigs of the same litter. In this particular case probably the very intensive contact of the IN vaccinated animals with the controls via the nipples of the sow caused the spread of vaccine virus to 1 of the control animals. This is the only case observed so far.

After IM or IN inoculation of piglets younger than 1 week the virus spread within the animal to various sites for up to 6 days after injection. The sites where vaccine virus has been found include brain, local lymph nodes, tonsils, lung, spleen and liver. Despite the viral spread within the very young animal, the piglets appeared completely healthy, and as shown above, no latency could be demonstrated. In a forced spreading experiment (also called back-passage) piglets younger than a week were inoculated with a high dose of vaccine by IM and IN routes. Nasal swabs were collected daily and pooled. In the second experiment also organ tissue homogenates were included in the consecutive inoculations. The results in Table 7 show that the vaccine virus disappeared in both experiments within 3 passages.

The last positive inoculum was amplified in tissue culture and given to a next couple of piglets. Virus recovered from the last passage had exactly the same characteristics as the initial inoculum: gI$^-$, TK$^-$ and avirulent.

TABLE 7 Virus titers during passages from piglet to piglet expressed as $TCID_{50}$/ml. The fifth inoculum is a repeated third passage after amplification of the virus in tissue culture.

Inoculum	Exp. 1	Exp. 2
1	6.4	8.3
2	2.6	5.1
3	1.4	3.2
4	<1.0	<1.0
5 (amplified)	7.4	6.6

Efficacy

In a series of 6 experiments the efficacy of the Begonia strain in protecting pigs against challenge with virulent field isolates has been demonstrated as shown in Tables 8 and 9.

The efficacy studies included a) challenge with 2 different strains: i.e. NIA-3 and 75V19, b) the use of seronegative specified pathogen free pigs, of commercially obtained seronegative pigs and of commercially obtained pigs with maternally derived antibody, c) a single and double IM vaccination procedure, and a single IN vaccination, and d) vaccinations between 4 and 12 weeks of age.

The most noteworthy result was that the efficacy study according to a standardized efficacy test described by De Leeuw and Van Oirschot (1985) showed that strain Begonia fully protected pigs against NIA-3 challenge, i.e. against the excretion of challenge virus and against growth retardation.

In the face of maternally-derived antibodies the efficacy results are less pronounced, but are well within the limits set by the European Pharmacopoeia (1987) for the efficacy of freeze-dried PRV vaccines in seronegative animals.

TABLE 8 Experimental design of efficacy studies

Exp.	1	2	3	4	5	6
Status of pig	MDA^- SPF	MDA^- SPF	MDA^+	MDA^+	MDA^+	MDA^+
No. of pigs vaccinated	4	8	8	8	10	9
No. of controls	4	8	8	8	5	5
Age at vacc (weeks)	7	7	8-10	8-10	10-12	10-12
Dose ($log_{10}TCID_{50}$)	5	5	4	4	5.5	5.5
Route	IM	IM	IM	IN	IM	2x IM
Time to challenge (weeks)	3	12	10	10	9	11
Challenge	NIA-3	NIA-3	75V19	75V19	75V19	75V19

MDA = maternally derived antibodies

TABLE 9 Summary of challenge results

Exp.	Vaccination Route	Average no. of days with: Growth retardation	Average no. of days with: Fever	Maximal duration of virus excretion (days)
1	1 x IM	5	2.5	not done
	—	13.5	5	not done
2	1 x IM	0	2	0
	—	13.5	8	4
3	1 x IM	6	5	8
	—	10	7	>14
4	1 x IN	5	4	8
	—	10	7	>14
5	1 x IM	8.5	3.5	7
	—	20	6	9
6	2 x IM	4	3	7
	—	20	6	>14

Experiences with strain Begonia in the field

In a controlled field trial with 176 fattening pigs, the animals were divided into 2 groups; 1 group received 1 IM vaccination, the other group 2 vaccinations with 2 weeks interval. In each pen 11 pigs were placed, of which at least 1 was left unvaccinated. Temperatures were recorded for 7 days and body weights for 5 weeks postvaccination. No significant differences between vaccinated animals and controls were observed. The efficacy of the immunization was tested in 5 animals of each group and found satisfactory as shown in Tables 8 and 9 (experiments 6 and 7). Until now over 1.5 million doses of strain Begonia have been used and no cases of adverse reactions were brought to our attention.

CONCLUSION

Pseudorabies virus vaccine strain Begonia complies with the original goal that the vaccine should pair high safety with a very strong immunogenicity.

ACKNOWLEDGEMENTS

We thank Dr. J.T. van Oirschot *et al.* for performing the initial tests, and Dr. H.J. Rziha for the hybridization experiments.

REFERENCES

European Pharmacopoeia, (draft version), 1987. Freeze-dried Aujeszky's disease live vaccine for pigs.

De Leeuw, P.W. and Van Oirschot, J.T. 1985. Vaccines against Aujeszky's disease: Evaluation of their efficacy under standardized laboratory conditions. Vet. Quarterly, **7,** 191-197.

Platt, K.B., Maré, C.J. and Hinz, P.N. 1979. Differentiation of vaccine strains and field isolates of pseudorabies virus: Thermal sensitivity and rabbit virulence markers. Archiv. Virol., **60,** 13-23.

Quint, W., Gielkens, A.L.J., Van Oirschot, J.T., Berns, A. and Cuypers, T.H. 1987. Construction and characterization of deletion mutants of pseudorabies virus: a new generation of live vaccines. J. Gen. Virol., **68,** 523-534.

SAFETY AND EFFICACY OF GENETICALLY ENGINEERED AUJESZKY'S DISEASE VACCINES

S. Kit

Division of Biochemical Virology
Baylor College of Medicine
Houston, Texas 77030, U.S.A.

ABSTRACT

Omnivac and Omnimark are modified-live pseudorabies vaccines derived from the Bucharest vaccine strain and have genetically engineered deletions in the thymidine kinase and thymidine kinase/glycoprotein g92 (gIII) genes, respectively. Omnivac has been used by American hog producers for 2.5 years with no adverse effects reported. Omnivac has also been employed to successfully eliminate Aujeszky's disease from quarantined farms. Extensive safety and efficacy studies on Omnimark have been completed in the U.S.A. and New Zealand in strict compliance with U.S.D.A. licensing procedures. These studies have shown that Omnimark: (1) is safe and effective in 3-day-old pigs; (2) is not transmitted from vaccinated animals to seronegative contact animals; (3) has not been isolated from the central nervous system or other tissues of vaccinated animals; (4) remains genetically stable following passage in pigs; (5) induces a serologic response in vaccinated pigs that allows differentiation between infected pigs and pigs vaccinated with other vaccines; and (6) is safe in a variety of laboratory animals.

INTRODUCTION

On January 20, 1986, Assistant Secretary of Agriculture Raymond D. Lett announced to representatives of the swine industry that the United States Department of Agriculture (U.S.D.A.) had licensed a novel pseudorabies vaccine, Omnivac, "the first recombinant-derived modified-live virus vaccine produced through biotechnology" (Lett, 1986). I will briefly describe some of the biochemical and biological properties of Omnivac. A second generation pseudorabies virus (PRV) vaccine, Omnimark, has also been produced in my laboratory (Kit, 1986; Kit *et al.*, 1986). Omnimark was derived from Omnivac by the deletion of a major glycoprotein gene, g92 (gIII), so that vaccinated pigs could be distinguished serologically from pigs infected with field strains of PRV. I will report on the biochemical and serological properties of Omnimark and safety and efficacy tests conducted with this virus in the United States and New Zealand. Finally, I will talk

J. T. van Oirschot (ed.), Vaccination and Control of Aujeszky's Disease, 45–55.

about the field experiences to date with Omnivac and the elimination of Aujeszky's disease (AD) from quarantined swine herds.

IN VITRO PROPERTIES OF OMNIVAC AND OMNIMARK

Omnivac was derived from a Bucharest strain of PRV which had been passaged over 800 times in chick cells and had been studied in the United States by Berger (Washington State University), Howarth (University of California at Davis), and Gustafson (Purdue University). Fig. 1 shows that the Kpn I and Bam HI restriction endonuclease patterns of the parental PRV strain, (BUK-O), received in Houston differed from that of the reference Aujeszky (Auj) strain of PRV in Kpn I-D, -E/F, and -I fragments and in Bam HI-7 and 12 fragments. The differences in the Bam Hi-7/12 and Kpn I-I fragments result from a 3.6 to 4.4 Kb deletion in the U_S + TR_S region of the genome of the Bucharest strain of PRV. Fig. 1 also shows that PRV (BUK-O)

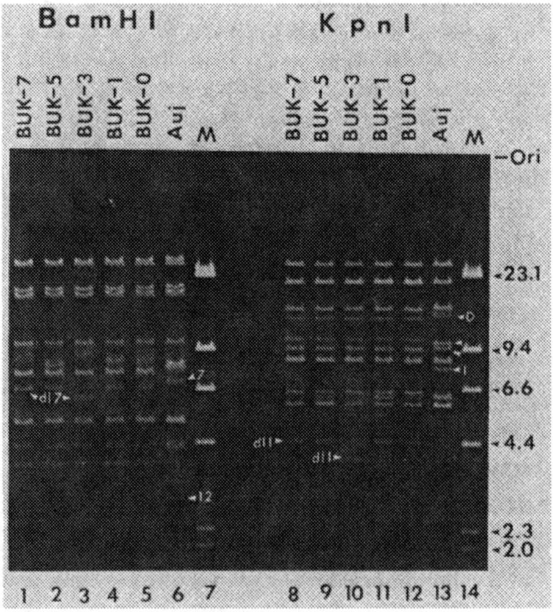

Fig. 1 Agarose gel electrophoresis analyses of DNA from PRV strains after cleavage with Bam HI and Kpn I. The PRV strains shown are Aujeszky (Auj) and the Bucharest (BUK-O) strain obtained from D.P. Gustafson (Purdue University). Bucharest clones 1, 3, 5, and 7 were plaque-purified from BUK-O. Lambda HindIII marker fragments are depicted in lanes 7 and 14 with the fragment sizes given in Kb. Ori = origin of electrophoresis.

consists of a mixture of at least 2 genotypes and that the Kpn I deletion in clone 3 of the Bucharest strain was greater than that in clones 1, 5, and 7.

To enhance the safety of the Bucharest strain, a 148 bp deletion and frame shift mutation was genetically engineered in the coding sequence of the thymidine kinase (TK) gene, thereby irreversibly inactivating this gene. The vaccine virus thereby obtained will be referred to as Omnivac or PRV (BUK-d13B) (Kit *et al.*, 1985b). Sequencing studies revealed that another genotypic characteristic distinguishing Omnivac from the Aujeszky strain of PRV was a 247 bp duplication in the Bam HI-11 fragment of Omnivac, but not of PRV (Auj) (Kit *et al.*, 1984).

Omnimark, or PRV (dlg92/dltk), the second generation vaccine virus, was produced from Omnivac by deleting a 1.1 Kb Sal I fragment from the major gIII gene of Omnivac. A "marker" vaccine strain was thereby obtained permitting the serological differentiation of vaccinated pigs from pigs infected with field strains (Kit *et al.*, 1987b).

To verify the TK-negative phenotype of Omnivac and Omnimark, TK enzyme assays, thymidine plaque autoradiography, and conventional autoradiographic studies on glass slides have been carried out. These experiments demonstrated that Omnivac and Omnimark do not express detectable TK activity. Further studies utilizing HAT selection techniques showed that Omnivac does not revert to the TK^+ phenotype, even under selective pressure.

To show that Omnimark did not induce the formation of glycoprotein gIII, immunoprecipitation experiments were performed on ^{3}H-mannose-labeled and ^{35}S-sulfate-labeled glycoproteins from virus-infected cells. Experiments were also carried out demonstrating that pigs vaccinated with Omnimark did not develop gIII antibodies, and that polyclonal or monoclonal antibodies against gIII did not immunoprecipitate gIII from extracts of gIII-negative, PRV-infected cells (Kit *et al.*, 1987a).

Plaque immunology experiments demonstrating the reaction of specific monoclonal antibodies to Omnimark and other PRV vaccine strains are shown in Table 1. The Bartha and our clone 3 Bucharest strains are gI-negative but gIII-positive, while Omnimark is gIII-negative and gI-positive.

Omnivac and Omnimark replicate and produce cytopathic effects in rabbit, porcine, bovine, murine, canine, feline, ovine, simian, hamster, and equine cells. Virus pools with titers in excess of 10^8 PFU/ml are routinely prepared after infection of subconfluent monolayer cultures of rabbit skin (RAB-9) or swine testicle (ST) cells for 3 days at 34.5°C or 39.1°C at an input multiplicity of about 0.01 to 0.03 PFU/cell. The vaccine dose used commercially is 10^5 $TCID_{50}$/ml. Thus, the titers of virus harvests are adequate for commercial production purposes.

TABLE 1 Plaque immunology demonstrating reaction of monoclonal antibodies with mutant PRV strains.

Virus strain	Specificity of monoclonal antibodies (MCA)			
	Anti-gII	Anti-gI	Anti-gIII	NMS**
Bartha	+*	—	+	—
BUK-C13	+	—	+	—
Omnimark	+	+	—	—
Mock-infected	—	—	—	—

* (+) and (—) = positive and negative staining plaques. MCA diluted 1:1000 and 1:2000. Plaques stained with peroxidase-labeled goat antibody to mouse IgG (H + L), chloronaphthol and peroxide.
** NMS = normal mouse ascites fluid.

The fact that a major portion of the PRV neutralizing antibody in swine sera is directed against gIII might suggest that a gIII-deleted vaccine virus cannot elicit a neutralizing antibody response. To investigate this possibility, rabbits, outbred and inbred mice, and swine were immunized with Omnimark, Omnivac, or the virulent PRV (P62/26) strain. Neutralizing antibodies were not found in nude mice. However, sera from Omnimark vaccinated pigs, rabbits, or mice equally neutralized the virulent PRV (P62/26) strain or Omnivac when measured by endpoint or plaque assay at high or low challenge virus titers (Dees *et al.*, 187; Kit *et al.*, 1987a).

ANIMAL STUDIES

Prior to licensing, the safety and efficacy of Omnivac was independently evaluated by E.C. Pirtle (U.S.D.A. National Animal Disease Center), Bruce Lawhorn (Texas A&M University), and Brad Thacker (Michigan State University). Omnimark is now in the final stages of the prelicensing process. Safety and efficacy studies on Omnimark have been independently conducted in mice, rabbits, hamsters, and guinea pigs by Craig Dees (Fermenta Animal Health), and in pigs by Bruce Lawhorn (Texas A&M University), Brad Thacker (Michigan State University), and R.W. Worthington (Ministry of Agriculture and Fisheries, New Zealand). The studies on mice demonstrated that intraperitoneal injection of Omnimark at $10^{7.5}$ $TCID_{50}$ per mouse did not kill outbred CFR, nude/nude, or beige mice (Kit *et al.*, 1987a). By contrast, commercial vaccines produced by Norden Laboratories and Pittmann-Moore killed 3 of 5 outbred mice in 7 days after intraperitoneal injection of

$10^{4.59}$ and $10^{3.59}$ $TCID_{50}$, respectively. Adverse reactions have not been observed after intracranial inoculation of Omnimark in pigs at 10^5 $TCID_{50}$, or after intramuscular (IM) inoculation of 3-day-old piglets at $10^{8.1}$ $TCID_{50}$. The IM inoculation of 10^5 $TCID_{50}$ in calves and lambs did not produce clinical signs of disease. Neither Omnivac nor Omnimark have been recovered from nasal swabs or from tissues after necropsy of pigs IM inoculated with virus. The vaccines protected pigs from severe intranasal (IN) challenge by virulent U.S.A. and New Zealand field strains and reduced shedding of challenge virus. Efforts to reisolate the challenge viruses from porcine tissues at necropsy have been unsuccessful.

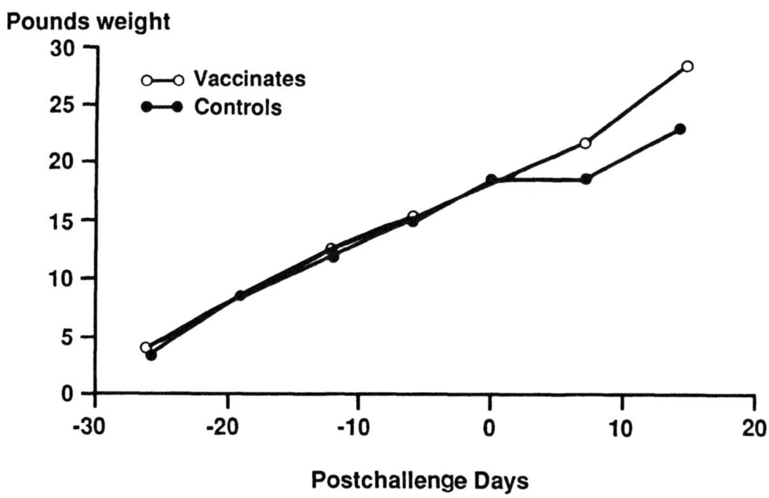

Fig. 2 Mean weight gains of vaccinated 3-day-old piglets and nonvaccinated controls.

The results of one of the safety and efficacy tests carried out on 3-day-old piglets by Fermenta Animal Health are shown in Figs. 2 and 3. Twenty piglets were IM vaccinated with 2ml ($10^{2.84}$) $TCID_{50}$ of Omnimark. Six littermates served as unvaccinated controls. At 26 days postvaccination, all piglets were IN challenged with the virulent PRV (P2208) strain at $10^{4.83}$ $TCID_{50}$ of virus. Piglets were bled 1 day prior to vaccination, at 7, 14, and 21 days postvaccination, and at 7 and 14 days postchallenge. The piglets were weighed on the day of vaccination, on 7, 14, and 21 days postvaccination, and at 0, 4, and 14 days postchallenge. Daily clinical observations were made for 14 days postchallenge, rectal temperatures were recorded, and nasal swabs were taken. At necropsy, virus isolation experiments were attempted on brain, liver, spleen, kidney, lung, and tonsil samples (Environmental Assessment and Finding of No Significant Impact for U.S.D.A.,

License, 1988).

At the time of vaccination, vaccinates and controls had average body weights of 3.9 and 3.6 pounds, respectively. On the day of challenge, vaccinates had gained an average of 14.2 pounds while the controls had gained an average of 14.9 pounds. For 7 days postchallenge, controls failed to gain weight and 4 of 6 controls died. During 14 postchallenge days, the vaccinated pigs gained 9.8 pounds, and the 2 surviving controls gained only 4.5 pounds (Fig. 2).

Postchallenge clinical signs, primarily of depression, were mild and transient in vaccinates. Neurological signs and mucous nasal discharge were not seen in any of the vaccinated piglets after challenge, while 5 of 6 nonvaccinated controls exhibited depression and 4 of 6 succumbed with severe neurological involvement. Of the 2 surviving controls, 1 showed depression, palor of the extremities, and was off feed, and the other control was off feed for 1 day.

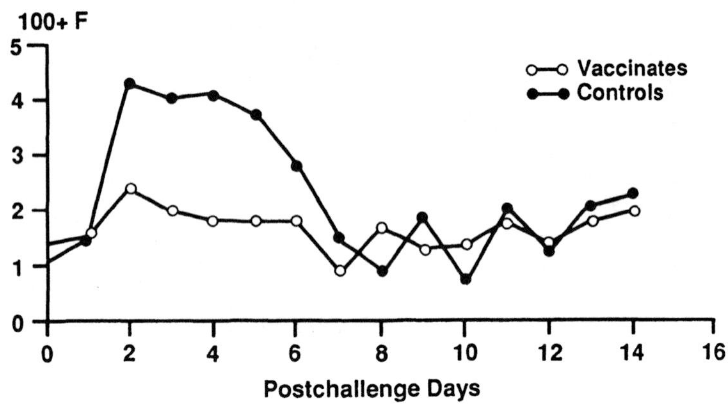

Fig. 3 Mean temperatures of vaccinated 1 to 3-day-old piglets and of nonvaccinated controls after challenge by virulent PRV (P2208).

Vaccinates and controls displayed a febrile response (> 103.0°F) over the 14-day postchallenge observation period (Fig. 3), but the temperature peaks of vaccinates were lower and more transient than in the controls and none of the vaccinates were pyrexic for more than 48 hr. However, 5 of the 6 controls were pyrexic from 3 to 5 days. Prior to vaccination, all piglets were seronegative to PRV. On the day of challenge (26 days postvaccination), all vaccinates had virus neutralization (VN) antibody titers of 1:8 or greater. Following challenge, all vaccinates showed an anamnestic response. All 6 nonvaccinated controls remained seronegative until challenge. Since the vaccinates and controls were housed together, the data indicate that there was no virus transmission from vaccinates to controls.

From 7 of 10 vaccinates, PRV was isolated in nasal swabs on either day 4 or 5 postchallenge and 1 piglet gave positive nasal swabs on both days 4 and 5. Four of 6 controls shed challenge virus for a minimum of 2 days with 3 controls shedding for 3 or more days.

PRV was not isolated from any of the tissues of vaccinated animals or from the 2 surviving controls following challenge, but PRV was isolated from the brain and tonsils of all the control pigs that succumbed to challenge and from the liver of 2 of the control pigs that died.

In the case of the New Zealand protection test, 6 pigs were IM vaccinated at 6 weeks and at 8 weeks of age with 2×10^7 $TCID_{50}$ of Omnimark (Oliver *et al.,* 1988). Two nonvaccinates served as contact controls. Nasal and tonsillar swabs were collected daily for 7 days postvaccination. All vaccinates and in-contact nonvaccinates remained healthy following vaccination and continued gaining weight. No pig became febrile. Virus was not isolated from nasal and tonsillar swabs of any of these pigs.

At 10 weeks of age, the above piglets and 4 age-matched piglets from the same source were challenge-inoculated IN with 2×10^7 $TCID_{50}$ of a PRV strain isolated from an outbreak of disease in New Zealand. Following challenge, all vaccinated pigs were febrile for 5 to 7 days but continued to gain weight, and all 6 vaccinates survived. Up to 5 to 7 days after challenge, PRV was isolated from nasal and tonsillar swabs. Substantial increases in serum antibody levels were detected 1 week after challenge. All nonvaccinated pigs died or became moribund within 6 days of challenge. Tonsil and nasal swabs were PRV-positive until the pigs died or became moribund. Isolations of PRV were made from one or more tissues of all nonvaccinates.

These vaccination trials show that Omnimark is safe and effective for vaccinating pigs against virulent U.S.A. and New Zealand isolates of PRV.

FIELD EXPERIENCE WITH OMNIVAC

In the 2.5 years since Omnivac was licensed, more than 1.5 million doses of Omnivac have been used without adverse effects. There have been no complaints by users to either the U.S.D.A. authorities or to the manufacturer. Omnivac has proven safe and effective in actual field use in 1 to 3-day-old piglets and in pregnant swine in all stages of gestation. The producers with large swine herds who enrolled in Omnivac vaccination/eradication programs include Atkinson Veterinary Service of Atkinson, Illinois, P-G Pork and Conhusker of Pilger, Nebraska, and Carrol Foods of Warsaw, North Carolina. Omnivac has been successfully used to eliminate AD from swine herds in Texas and in North Carolina.

With regard to the Texas study, an outbreak of AD occurred in February, 1984, in a breeding herd in Lometa, Texas following infection of sows by PRV-positive feral boars (Kit *et al.*, 1985a). The herd was quarantined. Slaughter of all 1,450 pigs on the farm was considered to prevent further spread of disease in Texas. As an alternative, the Texas Extension Veterinarians with the permission of the Texas State Animal Health Commissioner vaccinated the entire herd in June, 1984, with 10^7 $TCID_{50}$ of Omnivac. The herd included 128 pregnant females, 56 nonpregnant females, 224 nursery pigs, 7 boars, and over 1,000 grower-finisher pigs. VN antibody titers were determined on all breeding sows in July, August, September, and periodically thereafter. Pigs with titers of 1:16 of greater were slaughtered. Only seronegative gilts were used as replacements breeders.

On May 11, 1985, 240 breeding animals were tested. Of these, 53 vaccinated animals had titers of 1:2 to 1:4, 1 had a titer of 1:8, and 1 gilt, identified as a previously infected, vaccinated animal that was not sent to slaughter, had a titer of 1:16. It was removed. None of the unvaccinated pigs born from vaccinated mothers were seropositive. On August 1, 1985, 14 unvaccinated replacement gilts were seronegative. No identifiable adverse reactions had occurred in the herd, even though 1,450 doses of vaccine had been administered.

On May 23, 1986, almost 2 years after the vaccination, 220 blood samples were again obtained from the breeding herd by the Texas Animal Health Commission. One hundred and twelve of these were from previously vaccinated sows; the remaining ones were from unvaccinated replacement gilts. Sixteen of the previously vaccinated sows had VN antibody titers of 1:2, 3 had titers of 1:4, and all other pigs were seronegative. The 19 seropositive sows represented only 18% of residual responders, considering that only about half of the pigs tested responded serologically in the original vaccination. Thus, the data indicate that: (1) the vaccine had been effective in containing the field PRV, as evidenced by the effective clean-up of the herd; (2) the vaccine virus was not shed into the environment; and (3) contact transmission via recrudescence of latent virus from vaccinated pigs was not a factor on this farm. Transmission did not occur from vaccinated boars to the sows they impregnated, from the sows to their baby piglets, and from the unvaccinated "sentinel" piglets to other pigs on the farm.

The most recent serological tests were performed on June 16, 1988, on 4 sows and on 7 piglets from their litters that became ill (presumably due to a bacterial infection). These animals were seronegative for PRV. There have been no clinical signs of disease on this farm for 4 years. Another round of serological tests on breeders has been scheduled for the fall of 1988.

Successful elimination of AD by Omnivac vaccination on the Reeves farm in Farmville, North Carolina has also been reported (Reeves, 1988). The endemic nature of PRV in this swine herd was established through a serological survey in September of 1986 which showed that 25 out of 33 breeding pigs had VN antibody titers of 1:8 to 1:256, and 6 had titers of 1:4. Nine out of 16 finishing floor pigs, 3 to 6 months of age, exhibited titers of 1:8 to 1:32, and 15 out of 21 growers, 6 weeks to 3 months of age had titers of 1:4 or 1:8. The entire breeding herd and all finishing floor pigs were vaccinated and a routine vaccination schedule was instituted on pigs 1 to 3 days of age and again at 10 to 12 weeks of age (after maternal antibodies had declined). Replacement gilts were vaccinated at 6 months of age after demonstrating a seronegative status. A turnover of the breeding herd was instituted and all replacements purchased from seronegative herds were quarantined for 14 days and vaccinated. By 1988, the finishing floor herd had been converted into one in which no positive animals were determined. In this herd, the number of serologically positive pigs has been reduced in the face of a natural challenge. The PRV elimination program had a sound economic basis and the endemic status of the herd was overcome without depopulation and repopulation.

CONCLUDING COMMENTS

The previous results demonstrate that AD can be eliminated from swine herds by Omnivac vaccination programs, sound management and measurements to determine a rapid anamnestic response (or IgM formation). Obviously, elimination of disease can be facilitated by safe and effective marker vaccines, such as Omnimark, which permit the producers to distinguish vaccinated animals from those infected by virulent field strains. The Omnimark vaccine has potential for use: (1) in vaccination in the face of an outbreak to protect pigs and prevent or limit the spread of virulent virus; (2) for large scale immunization/eradication programs where test and slaughter procedures are too costly or logistically difficult to mount or sustain; (3) for removing the quarantine stigma from an infected herd; and (4) to reduce the hazards of moving pigs carrying latent PRV infections across state and national boundaries. The data presented in Table 2 illustrate the feasibility of tests to differentiate gIII-positive from gIII-negative sera. It may be seen that sera with VN antibody titers of 1:4 or greater from field infections or from pigs immunized with gIII-positive viruses give positive plaque immunology tests on plaques formed by PRV (Auj) and on plaques formed by a genetically engineered marmoset herpesvirus (MarHV) strain that expresses the PRV glycoprotein gIII, but not on plaques formed by the parental MarHV. PRV antibodies in sera from pigs vaccinated with Omnimark detected plaques formed by PRV (Auj), but not MarHV (Prg92) or MarHV. A commercial diagnostic test based upon competition of field sera with peroxidase-conjugated, anti gIII-specific monoclonal antibodies has been developed by Fermenta Animal Health and will be available as a companion kit with the Omnimark vaccine.

TABLE 2 Antibodies to PRV gIII in sera of infected herds detected by plaque immunology*

		gIII-Positive plaques from:		
Sera and Source	VN titer	PRV(Auj)	MarHV (gIII)	MarHV**
1 Ill. Dept. Ag.	1:4	+	+	—
2 Ill. Dept. Ag.	1:8	+	+	—
3 Ill. Dept. Ag.	1:16	+	+	—
4 Ill. Dept. Ag.	1:32	+	+	—
5 Omnivac Maddox	1:4	+	+	—
6 Omnivac Maddox	1:8	+	+	—
7 Omnimark Vacc1	1:4	+	—	—
8 Omnimark Vacc2	ND	+	—	—
9 E.C. Pirtle	1:256	+	+	—
0 Ill. Dept. Ag.	Neg	—	—	—

* Plaques on RAB-9 cells detected by biotin-rabbit anti-porcine IgG (H + L), peroxidase-conjugated streptavidine, chloronaphthol and hydrogen peroxide. Sera were serially diluted from 1:256 to 1:16384.

** MarHV = marmoset herpesvirus. MarHV (gIII) = a recombinant MarHV expressing the PRV gIII protein.

REFERENCES

Dees, C., Bartkoski, M. and Kit, S. 1987. Neutralization of Omnivac-PRV and PRV (dlg92 / dltk. Abstracts of papers presented at the Conference of Research Workers on Animal Diseases (Nov. 16-17, 1987; Chicago, Illinois). p. 338.

Environmental Assessment and Finding of No Significant Impact for U.S.D.A. License issued by U.S.D.A.-A.P.H.I.S. to Fermenta Animal Health, 1988.

Kit, S. 1986. Vaccinated pigs can be distinguished serologically from field-strain infected pigs. In "Official Proceedings of the 1986 Annual Meeting of the Livestock Conservation Institute" (Omaha, Nebraska). pp. 120-123.

Kit, S., Kit, M., Bartkoski, M.J. and Dees, C. 1987a. Genetically engineered pseudorabies vaccine with deletions in thymidine kinase and glycoprotein genes. In "Vaccines 87. Modern Approaches to New Vaccines: Prevention of AIDS and Other Viral, Bacterial, and Parasitic Diseases" (Eds. R.M. Chanock, R.A. Lerner, F. Brown and H. Ginsberg). (Cold Spring Harbor Laboratory, N.Y.). pp. 345-348.

Kit, S., Kit, M., Lawhorn, B. and McConnell, S. 1985a. Immunization of pregnant pigs in a quarantined swine herd with a thymidine kinase deletion mutant of pseudorabies virus. In "High Technology Route to Virus Vaccines" (Eds. G.R. Dreesman, J.G. Bronson and R.C. Kennedy). (American Society for Microbiology, Washington, D.C.). pp. 82-99.

Kit, S., Kit, M. and Otsuka, H. 1984. Structure of viral thymidine kineases. In "Herpesviruses" (Ed. F. Rapp). (Alan R. Liss, Inc., N.Y.). pp. 311-327.

Kit, S., Kit, M. and Pirtle, E.C. 1985b. Attenuated properties of thymidine kinase-negative deletion mutant of pseudorabies virus. Am. J. Vet. Res., **46,** 1359-1367.

Kit, S., Sheppard, M., Ichimura, H. and Kit, M. 1987b. Second-generation pseudorabies virus vaccine with deletions in thymidine kinase and glycoprotein genes. Am. J. Vet. Res., **48,** 780-793.

Kit, S., Sheppard, M. and Kit, M. 1986. Control of Aujeszky's disease. Vet. Rec., **118,** 310.

Lett, R.D. 1986. U.S.D.A. philosophy of livestock disease control and eradication. In "Proceedings of the PRV Symposium: Following Upon the Pilot Projects What Next?" (Published by the National Pork Producer's Council, Des Moines, Iowa). pp. 20-25.

Oliver, R.E., Motha, M.J.X., Worthington, R.W., Penrose, M.E. and Poole, W.S. 1988. Protection of piglets against a virulent New Zealand isolate of Aujeszky's disease virus by vaccination with a novel genetically engineered vaccine. New Zealand Vet. J. (in press).

Reeves, D.E. 1988. Results of a field study using a genetically altered modified live pseudorabies vaccine in an eradication program. In "Proceedings of the Annual Meeting of the American Association of Swine Practitioners" (March 6-8, 1988, St. Louis, Missouri). pp. 263-264.

SUMMARY

The first paper by Mettenleiter dealt with an analysis of the factors that affect virulence of pseudorabies virus (PRV). The salient findings of the results showed that several different PRV gene products can affect virulence. Elimination of one of these gene products (with the exception of the thymidine kinase) does not necessarily affect virulence; a combination of defects in these genes abolishes virulence without necessarily affecting the ability of the virus to grow in cell culture. Thus, mutations in these genes affect virulence synergistically.

The second paper, by Post, set the stage for the description of the thymidine kinase (TK) minus/gX minus (Tolvid) vaccine which was subsequently discussed by Wardley. Post described the characteristics of the gX protein. This protein is synthesized as a cell bound precursor and is then released from the cells. The fact that this glycoprotein is nonessential for virus growth in cell culture, that it is highly immunogenic but that immunization with this glycoprotein does not protect against challenge with virulent virus, indicates that it may be a good candidate for deletion from a vaccine strain, thereby allowing differentiation by serological means between vaccinated pigs and pigs that have also been exposed to wild type strains of PRV.

The next 4 papers concerned the characterizations of the efficacy and safety of genetically engineered live vaccines of PRV. All the vaccines described were TK^- (to render them avirulent) and were defective in the synthesis of one nonessential viral glycoprotein which was either gX (strain Tolvid; Post and Wardley), gI (strains Begonia and 783; Lütticken and Gielkens) or gIII (strain Omnimark; Kit). The 4 papers dealt with experiments in which the ability of the vaccines to prevent disease, animal weight loss, as well as excretion of virus after superinfection with virulent virus was tested. In general, the vaccines were found to be effective and safe in pigs at the doses of vaccine and of challenge virus used. The vaccines were also shown to be innocuous for either other farm animals, laboratory animals or pet animals.

Other noteworthy observations that were reported were as follows: 1. Wardley showed that a TK^- vaccine that is also gI^-/gX^- is less protective than is a vaccine that is TK^- and gX^- only, indicating either that deletion of gI renders the vaccine strain less protective than deletion of gX or that deletion of both gI and gX have a synergistic effect on vaccine efficacy. 2. Wardley showed that the TK^-/gX^- (Tolvid) vaccine is more effective in preventing excretion of superinfecting virulent virus than is the Pr-Vac (Norden) vaccine. He also reported that infection of animals with a mixture of the Tolvid and Pr-Vac vaccines did not result in the emergence of virulent recombinants. 3. Lütticken reported that the TK^-/gI^- (Begonia) vaccine has been

J. T. van Oirschot (ed.), Vaccination and Control of Aujeszky's Disease, 57–58.

extensively used in the field without any adverse reaction. 4. Kit reported that the BUK TK^- (Omnivac) vaccine has been successfully used to eliminate PRV from quarantined farms.

Although all the vaccines described where shown to be safe and effective, the comparison of the relative efficacy of the 4 vaccines that were described to those of other vaccines that have been marketed for years, was not possible on the basis of the results presented because different doses of regimens of vaccination, different doses of challenge, different strains of challenge virus, different age animals, etc. were used.

It is clear that a vaccine should not only prevent disease but should also prevent establishment of latency by a superinfecting virulent strain, thereby eliminating the virus reservoir. Presumably, the more immunogenic the vaccine, the more likely it will be to prevent establishment of latency. The question as to which vaccine is the more immunogenic is therefore of considerable significance. The role of the nonessential glycoproteins that are deleted from each of the vaccines in the ability of the virus to replicate in the vaccinated animals or their direct role in the immune response needs to be investigated to ascertain which of these glycoproteins can be deleted with the least effect on the efficacy of the vaccine.

2. NEW DEVELOPMENTS IN AUJESZKY'S DISEASE VACCINES

Chairpersons H.J. Rziha and B. Lomniczi

CONSTRUCTION OF A RECOMBINANT ADENOVIRUS WHICH EXPRESSES THE PSEUDORABIES VIRUS gp50: PRELIMINARY RESULTS

M. Eloit, M. Perricaudet**, B. Toma**

*Institut National de la Recherche Agronomique
Laboratoire d'Epidémiologie et de physiopathologie des maladies á virus
E.N.V. Alfort, 94704 Maison-Alfort Cedex, France
**Centre National de la Recherche Scientifique
Institut Gustave Roussy, 94800 Villejuif, France

ABSTRACT

The aim of this work was to construct a recombinant adenovirus which could express the gp50 gene of pseudorabies virus and to test it as a vaccine in different animal species. As a preliminary work, we have constructed a recombinant plasmid which harbors the very left end of adenovirus type 5 and the gp50 gene of pseudorabies virus under the control of the adenovirus major late promoter. This plasmid was shown by immunofluorescence to direct the synthesis of gp50 in a transient expression assay. For the construction of the recombinant adenovirus, the very left end of the adenovirus type 5 genome will be replaced by viral sequences carried by the plasmid.

INTRODUCTION

Besides poxvirus-based vectors, whose suitability for in vivo expression of foreign genes is now well demonstrated, several other virus families (adenoviridae, herpesviridae) are candidate to be used as viral vectors in vaccination of animals. Among these viruses, the potential use of adenovirus type 5 (Ad5) as gene transfer vector is based on different arguments: its genetic organization has been widely studied; different deletion mutants, with insertion capacity of up to 7 kbp, have been isolated and can be propagated in Ad-transformed human cell lines, like 293 cells; the high copy number of genome in infected cells and the strength of some viral promoters lead to the synthesis of large amounts of viral products during replication; furthermore, Ad5 seems to have a wide host range and has been shown to replicate in man, rabbit (Ballay *et al.*, 1985, 1987), hamster (Morin *et al.*, 1987), mouse (Johson *et al.*, 1987) and pig (Betts *et al.*, 1962). Recombinant Ad5 harboring hepatitis B surface antigen gene was capable of inducing antibodies against

J. T. van Oirschot (ed.), Vaccination and Control of Aujeszky's Disease, 61–66.

hepatitis B surface antigen in rabbits and mice (Ballay *et al.*, 1985, 1987); Johson *et al.*, 1987), and to protect chimpanzees from virulent challenge (Levrero *et al.*, 1987). To test the suitability of Ad5 as an in vivo gene transfer vector in several animal species, it appeared necessary to use a model which could permit easy and fast virulent challenges in a wide range of host species. Pseudorabies virus was chosen on this criterion, and because of its economical importance in the swine industry.

Among the different glycoproteins of pseudorabies virus (PRV), gp50 seems to be a good candidate to incorporate in a subunit vaccine. Wathen *et al.* (1985) first demonstrated that gp50 was a target of neutralizing monoclonal antibodies which can protect mice against the sequelae of PRV challenge. We recently extended these findings by showing that gp50 was the only protein recognized by neutralizing monoclonal antibodies derived from a fusion using live virus as immunogen (Eloit *et al.*, 1988). Furthermore, gp50 delivered either to mice via infection by a recombinant vaccinia virus, or to pig as a protein produced in CHO cells, was shown to protect against PRV-induced disease (Marchioli *et al.*, 1987).

We describe in this report the transient expression in a human cell line of the open reading frame coding for gp50 (Petrovskis *et al.*, 1986), under the control of the major late promoter (MLP) of adenovirus type 2 (Ad2). Immunofluorescence analysis showed that the gp50 produced was mainly membrane-associated.

MATERIALS AND METHODS

Materials

Restriction enzymes, T4 DNA ligase and E. coli DNA polymerase (Klenow fragment) were purchased from Boehringer Mannheim and Bethesda Research Laboratories.

Cells

The 293 cell line is an adenovirus transformed human embryonic cell line which was maintained in Dulbecco's modified Eagle medium (DMEM) containing 10% fetal calf serum (FCS).

Plasmids

The plasmid pPRVB7 which contains the BamHI fragment no. 7 of the NIA3 PRV strain, cloned at the unique BamHI site of pBR322, is a gift of Gila Kohen (Rhône Mérieux, Lyon, France).

The eukaryotic expression vector pMLP10 has already been described (Ballay *et al.*, 1987). This plasmid contains an association of the very left-end of the Ad5 genome and of the MLP of Ad2 joined to its tripartite leader sequence. pMLP10/CAT is a gift of Dominique Brechemier Baey (Institut Gustave Roussy, Villejuif, France). It contains the CAT gene followed by splicing (nucleotides 4099-4705) and polyadenylation signals (nucleotides 2553-2770) from SV40, cloned downstream the MLP and its tripartite leader sequence.

Plasmid DNAs were prepared according to the method of Birnboim and Doly (1979) followed by 2 cesium chloride-ethidium bromide equilibrium gradient centrifugations.

Monoclonal Antibodies

Production and characterization of anti-gp50 monoclonal antibodies have been described (Eloit *et al.*, 1988).

Cell transfection and immunofluorescence assay

293 cells were transfected with 5μg of plasmid DNA and 5 μg of salmon sperm carrier DNA, by the calcium phosphate method (Graham and Van der Eb, 1973). pMLP10 CAT was used as a negative control. Two days later, cells were fixed by ethanol for 15 min at room temperature. A mix of 3 different anti-gp50 monoclonal antibodies (22M24, 2T22, 41Y10) was used to probe the fixed cells (1 hour, 37°C). After 3 washes with phosphate buffered saline, bound antibodies were revealed with an antimouse serum labelled with fluorescein (Amersham).

Labelling of gp50 and immunoprecipitation

Twenty-four hours after transfection, DMEM was replaced with Eagle's minimal essential medium plus 10 μCi of ^{14}C glucosamine per ml. Twenty-four hours later, the cells were lysed by 0.05 M Tris, 0.5M NaCl, 1% Triton X100, sodium deoxycholate 0.1%, ovalbumine 1 mg/ml, SDS 0.1%. The method of immunoprecipitation has been described (Eloit *et al.*, 1988).

RESULTS AND DISCUSSION

Construction of plasmid pMLP10gp50.6

The NdeI-Stu I fragment of pPRVB7 was cloned between NdeI and HindIII sites of pBR322, after filling in the HindIII end with Klenow, to give plasmid pPRVSN. This was done to eliminate some undesirable NarI sites upstream and downstream the gp50 gene. The construction of the expression vector used the NarI site 36 base-pairs upstream the translation initiation signal and the MaeIII site 47 base-pairs downstream the translation stop signal. Partial NarI digestion and MaeIII digestion of pPRVSN gave a 1287bp fragment which contains the whole coding sequence of gp50. After filling in the MaeIII end with Klenow, this fragment was inserted between ClaI and HpaI sites of pMLP10/CAT to give pMLP10/gp50.6, in which the SV40 polyadenylation signal just follows the gp50 coding sequence without any splicing signals. A ClaI site, necessary for the construction of the recombinant adenovirus, was created by digesting the unique BamHI site of pMLP10/gp50.6, filling in the ends with Klenow and religating (Fig. 1).

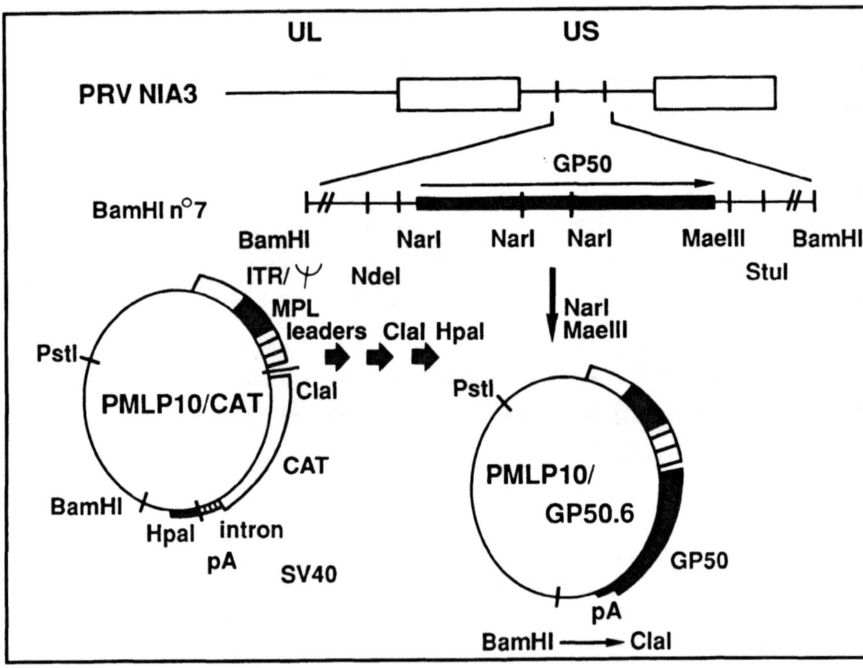

Fig. 1 Construction of the pMLP10/gp50.6 plasmid. The NarI-MaeIII fragment of PRV BamHI-7 DNA was inserted between the ClaI and HpaI sites of pMLP10/CAT.

Transfection of the pMLP10/gp50.6 plasmid into 293 cells

The ability of pMLP10/gp50.6 to direct the synthesis of gp50 was tested in a transient expression assay after transfection of 293 cells. The gp50 expression was analyzed by an immunofluorescence assay using a mix of 3 anti-gp50 monoclonal antibodies. A mix of monoclonal antibodies was preferred to the use of 1 monoclonal antibody to take into account the risk of non-expression of a particular epitope. As shown in Fig. 2, a protein was recognized in cells transfected with pMLP10/gp50.6 and not in cells transfected with the negative control (pMLP10/CAT). This protein was mainly membrane-associated. As the coding sequence we cloned was previously shown to direct the synthesis of gp50 (Marchioli *et al.*, 1987), and because of the specificity of the monoclonal antibodies used to probe the transfected cells, we assume that the recognized protein is gp50. Immunoprecipitation experiments showed that the produced protein had the same molecular weight as gp50 synthesized in PRV infected 293 cells (data not shown).

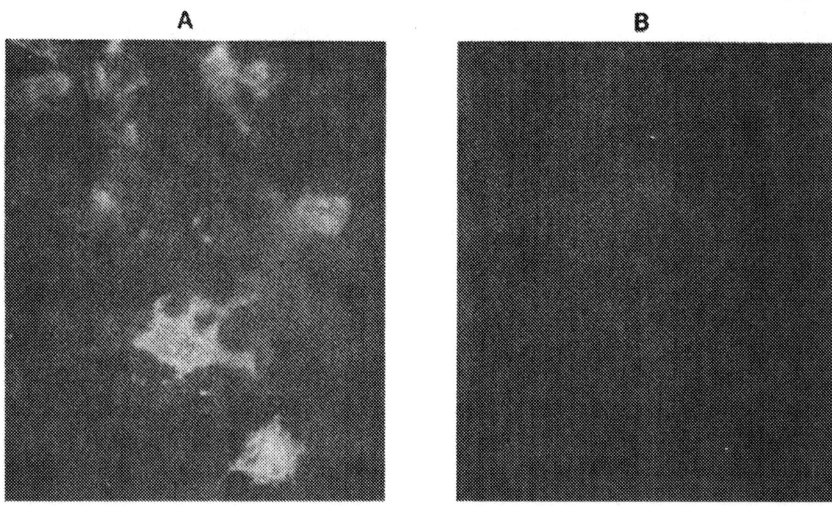

Fig. 2 The 293 cell line were transfected with pMLP10/gp50.6 (A), or pMLP10/CAT as negative control (B). Immunofluorescence assay was conducted with anti-gp50 monoclonal antibodies.

CONCLUSION

We have constructed a recombinant plasmid which harbors the very left-end of Ad5 and the gp50 gene of PRV under the control of the adenovirus MLP. This plasmid was shown to direct the synthesis of gp50 in a transient expression assay. As described by Ballay *et al.* (1987), this plasmid will be used to replace in vitro the very left-end of the Ad5 genome by the PstI-ClaI fragment of the recombinant plasmid. The recombinant adenovirus will be tested as a potential vaccine in different animal species.

ACKNOWLEDGEMENTS

We thank Mrs. A. Fournier and M. Adam for their excellent technical assistance and Mrs. P. Gilardi, I. Joab and E. Tosoni-Pitoni for helpful advice.

REFERENCES

Ballay, A., Levrero, M., Buendia, M.A., Tiollais, P. and Perricaudet, M. 1985. In vitro and in vivo synthesis of the hepatitis B surface antigen and of the receptor for polymerised human serum albumin from recombinant human adenoviruses. EMBO, **4**, 3861-3865

Ballay, A., Levrero, M., Tiollais, P. and Perricaudet, M. 1987. An Hepatitis B adenovirus recombinant as a potential live vaccine in Hepadnaviruses. UCLA symposia on molecular and cellular biology, New Series, Vol. **70**. (Eds. W. Robinson, K. Koike and H. Will). (Alan R. Liss Inc, New York). pp.481-493.

Betts, A.O., Jennings, A.R., Lamont, P.H. and Page, Z. 1962. Inoculation of pigs with adenoviruses of man. Nature, **193**, 45-46.

Birnboim, H.C. and Doly, J. 1979. A rapid extraction procedure for screening recombinant plasmid DNA. Nucl. Acids. Res., **7**, 1513-1523.

Eloit, M., Fargaud, D., L'Haridon, R. and Toma, B. 1988. Identification of the pseudorabies glycoprotein gp50 as a major target of neutralizing antibodies. Arch. Virol., **99**, 45-56.

Graham, F.L. and Van der Eb, A.J. 1973. A new technique for the assay of infectivity of human Adenovirus 5 DNA. Virology, **52**, 456-467.

Johson, D.C., McDermott, M.R., Choudhury, G.G. and Graham, F.L. 1987. Cells infected with an adenovirus vector express very high levels of HSV. 1 gB and become clumped and extensively vacuolated. Proceedings of the 12th international herpesvirus workshop, University of Pennsylvania, Philadelphia. p. 161.

Levrero, M., Ballay, A., Schellekens, H., Tiollais, P. and Perricaudet, M. 1987. Live recombinant adenovirus can protect chimpanzee against Hepatitis B, in Proceedings of the Basic Vaccinology Meeting, dec. 1987, Geneva, Switzerland.

Marchioli, C.C., Yancey, R.J., Petrovskis, E.A., Timmins, J.G. and Post, L.E. 1987. Evaluation of pseudorabies virus glycoprotein gp50 as a vaccine for Aujeszky's disease in mice and swine: expression by vaccinia virus and chinese hamster ovary cells. J. Virol., **61**, 3977-3982.

Morin, J.E., Lubeck, M.P., Barton, J.E., Conley, A.J., Davis, A.R. and Hung, P.P. 1987. Recombinant adenovirus induces antibody response to Hepatitis B virus surface antigen in hamsters. Proc. Natl. Acad. Sci. U.S.A., **84**, 4626-4630.

Petrovskis, E.A., Timmins, J.G., Armentrout, M.A., Marchioli, C.C., Yancey, R.J. and Post, L.E. 1986. DNA sequence of the gene for pseudorabies virus gp50, a glycoprotein without N-linked glycosylation. J. Virol., **59**, 216-223.

Wathen, L.M.K., Platt, K.B., Wathen, M.W., Van Densen, R.A., Whestone, C.A. and Pirtle, E.C. 1985. Production and characterization of monoclonal antibody directed against pseudorabies virus. Virus Res., **4**, 19-29.

INDUSTRIAL PRODUCTION AND CONTROL OF A SUBUNIT VACCINE AGAINST AUJESZKY'S DISEASE

G. Chappuis, D. Fargeaud, A. Brun

Rhône Mérieux
Laboratoire IFFA
254, rue Marcel Mérieux
69007 Lyon, France

ABSTRACT

This paper presents the methods used for the preparation and control of a viral subunit vaccine: Geskypur.[1] This vaccine is an industrial vaccine of which several million doses have already been administered. We shall emphasize some parameters relative to tests done during the manufacturing process (purity, identity, envelope glycoprotein content) and potency tests performed in the porcine, canine and feline species. At the end of the paper, we shall consider the problem posed by the possibility of distinguishing between convalescent pigs and vaccinated pigs. This vaccine is of a totally original conception and represents an important and interesting technological advance in the field of herpesviruses and for the medical control of herpesvirus infections.

INTRODUCTION

Vaccination against human or animal herpesvirus infections with traditional live or inactivated vaccines had posed problems of safety and/or efficacy. With regard to Aujeszky's disease (AD), the wide-scale use of an inactivated, crude killed virus based vaccine containing an oil emulsion as adjuvant has lead to the observation, in certain farms, of postvaccinal allergic-type reactions, such as lack of appetite or hyperthermia, or, more serious reactions, such as abortion in pregnant sows. The analysis of these phenomena lead to the conclusion that they always occurred in animals which had developed "sensitivity" to pseudorabies virus (PRV) during convalescence or following vaccination. Because this type of incident, its analysis and its solution had initially been treated for the Feline herpesvirus (FHV) (Chappuis *et al.*, 1981), we applied the same process to PRV. The research work consisted in developing a technique to extract the immunogenic viral glycoproteins. This process had to be applicable at an industrial level, economically viable and lead to the

[1] Rhône Mérieux Trademark

J. T. van Oirschot (ed.), Vaccination and Control of Aujeszky's Disease, 67–78.

preparation of a purified vaccine as safe and active as possible.

After describing the process of preparation of the Geskypur vaccine, we shall present the advantages that this original vaccine has compared to conventional vaccines, particularly due to its purity and the level of standardization both of its formula and of its potency tests by virulent challenge in the target species. Since immunogenic viral fractions are used and the capsid fractions are excluded, we were able to consider differentiation between vaccinated animals and infected animals. This objective was achieved by the use of immunogenic fractions from a viral strain deleted in glycoprotein I (gI).

PRODUCTION METHOD OF THE SUBUNIT VACCINE

Viral strain

In an initial stage, the first batches of vaccine were prepared from the Kojnok strain of PRV. This prototype virulent strain did not contain any deletions, and was subsequently replaced by the KaH strain (Mettenleiter *et al.*, 1987) from Vanderbilt University, Nashville, USA, kindly provided by Dr. Ben-Porat. The KaH strain carries deletions in genes encoding gI and gp63, which meant that by testing for the corresponding antibodies, vaccinated pigs could be differentiated from infected pigs.

Cells

The BHK_{21} cell line is used, and cultured in suspension in 1000 to 2800 liters fermentor vessels in Stocker's medium containing 10% calf serum.

Culture and inactivation

During the viral cycle, temperature is maintained at 37°C. The viral suspension is inactivated by adding ethyleneimine at a concentration of 0.5 per 1000.

Purification of the viral glycoproteins

The inactivated viral suspension is concentrated by ultrafiltration. The clarified concentrate is purified in 2 steps: by polyethylene glycol precipitation and by rate-zonal ultracentrifugation. The viral envelope containing the glycoproteins is dissociated from the capsid by addition of polyoxyethylene alcohol. The viral capsids are discarded by ultracentrifugation. The supernatant represents the concentrated solution of purified glycoproteins which is stored, deep frozen at -40°C.

Preparation of the actual vaccine

The concentrated solution of glycoproteins is thawed and diluted in a pH 7.8 phosphate buffer, so that the glycoprotein content is adjusted to 10μg/dose. The diluted solution of glycoproteins is blended, under strong agitation, to the oil excipient to obtain an emulsion. The emulsion is then cooled to 4°C. It is obvious that numerous tests are performed throughout the entire manufacturing period on the raw materials (viral and cell strains, and media) and also on the viral antigen from the pre-inactivation crude virus stage through to the glycoprotein subunits.

Study of some parameters related to production

Industrialization: The down stream processing leads to large batches of product, the formulation of which is perfectly standardized. The process leads to reproducible and economically viable performances.

Identity and purity of glycoprotein viral subunits. Qualitative aspect: The separation of viral polypeptides by polyacrylamide gel electrophoresis, under reducing and non-reducing conditions, provides a way to identify and test the purity of the viral glycoproteins by a combination of 2 revelation methods (Hampl *et al.*, 1984). An initial step using fluorochrome-labelled lectin only reveals the glycoproteins (due to their glucidic residues). Under non reducing conditions the 2 major glycoproteins - the gII and gIII complex and, to a lesser extent, the minor glycoprotein gp50 (Fargeaud *et al.*, 1984) are identified by fluorescence. Under reducing conditions, 4 major fluorescent bands are visible, which represent gIIa, gIII, gIIb and gIIc (Fig. 1).

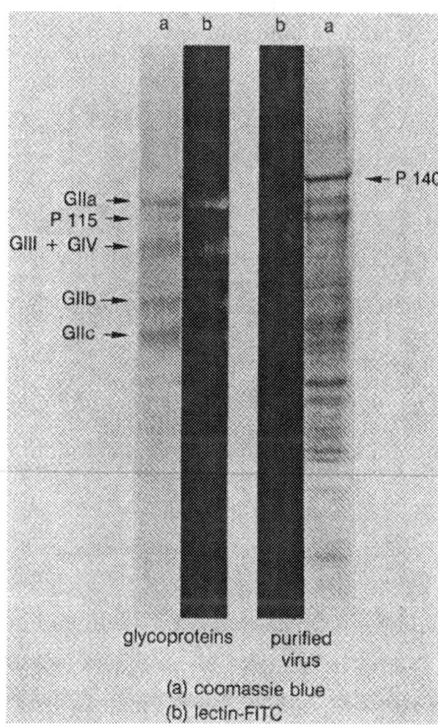

Fig. 1 Polyacrylamide gel electrophoresis of purified PRV and glycoprotein solution

Any other fluorescent band is the sign of a lesser degree of purity. This first step is followed by a second one, which consists of the staining of all proteins with Coomassie's Blue; this stain, which identifies all the viral polypeptides, is a measure of the purity of the preparation by showing that no bands other than glycoproteins are present.

Quantitative evaluation of viral proteins in the glycoprotein solution following purification: The proteins are precipitated using trichloracetic acid in the presence of deoxycholate and assayed using Folin's reagent. The concentration in total proteins is established by comparison with a range of bovine albumin.

Quantitative evaluation of the major glycoproteins gII and gIII: As the 2 major glycoproteins have no antigenic relationship, they are evaluated separately by radial immunodiffusion. This technique is carried out by placing dilutions of the glycoprotein preparation in the wells of an agar plate containing sheep serum specifically directed against one of the glycoproteins. The presence of precipitation rings after diffusion is a proof of identity. The quantitative evaluation is obtained by comparing the size of the rings with those of a glycoprotein reference solution (Fig. 2).

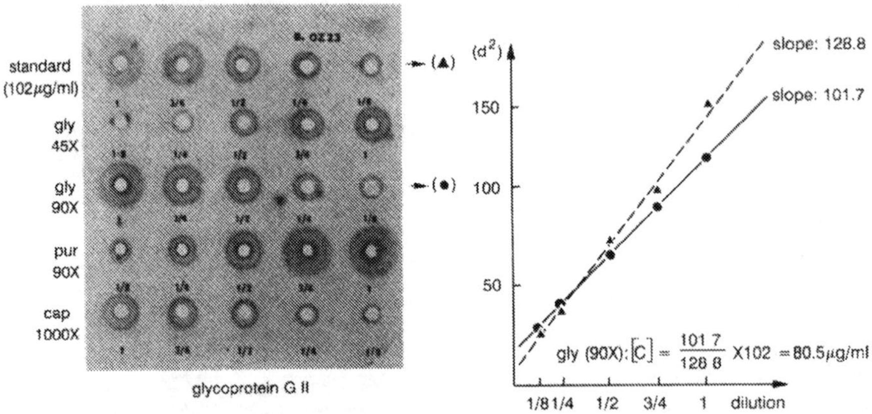

Fig. 2 **Single radial immunodiffusion evaluation of PRV glycoproteins.**

The glycoprotein content measured in the concentrated solution is then used to prepare the vaccinal antigenic solution by dilution and adjustment of its glycoprotein concentration to 10 µg/dose (gII + gIII). Table 1 presents results of productivity in overall glycoproteins of several industrial harvests of varying volumes. Variations in glycoprotein yields should be noted.

TABLE 1 Glycoprotein productivity results from several industrial harvests

Culture no.	Volume (liters)	Pre-inactivation infective titer (log_{10}/ml)	Quantity of glycoproteins (mg) *
OAO1	950	9.0	5912
OEO5	800	9.2	8267
OGO7	940	8.4	3216
OHO8	1000	7.1	723
OIO9	990	7.6	1199
OK10	990	8.5	4698
OL11	970	8.5	5005
OM12	976	8.9	4530
OP15	933	9.3	2058
OS16	980	8.9	3998
OT17	980	8.9	4787
OV19	1300	9.2	1927
OZ23	1000	8.9	2883
OC26	980	8.9	6702
OF29	2200	9.1	9580
OJ32	2780	9.4	12652
OK33	970	9.2	6915

* x 100 = number of doses/batch

TABLE 2 Results of gII and gIII assays in several industrial batches of concentrated antigen

Batches of concentrated antigen	Proteins μg/ml	Glycoproteins gII (μg/ml)	Glycoproteins gIII(μg/ml)
OGO7	976	225.1	333.7
OK10	890	459.6	411.3
OL11	1934	472.3	545.3
OR15	488	118.0	267.4
OS16	1323	448.8	772.2
OW20	670	265.3	347.2
OZ23	912	231.1	298.9
OB25	738	296.5	396.2
OD27	616	174.6	262.8
OG30	671	154.7	274.0
OH31	959	310.6	353.2

Table 2 presents the quantitative evaluation of gII and gIII in several industrial batches of concentrated antigen.

Fig. 3 shows the amounts of total proteins and viral glycoproteins during the different steps of purification.

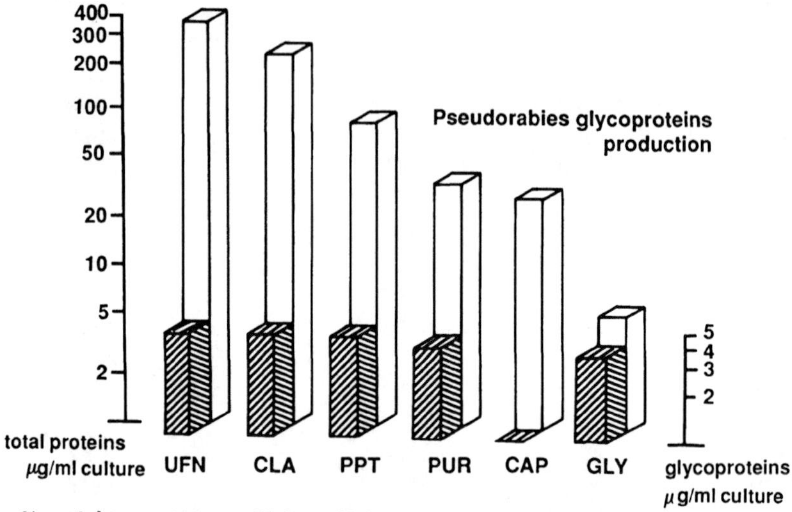

	UFN	CLA	PPT	PUR	CAP	GLY
% proteins	100	65.8	23.3	9.5	8.2	1.4
%glycoproteins/ proteins	1.2	1.8	5.2	10.9	1.0	66.7

Fig. 3 Concentrations of proteins and glycoproteins along the down stream processing. For abbreviations see text.

It should be noted that after ultrafiltration (UFN), the viral glycoprotein level represents 1.2% of the total proteins, and that the purification steps (CLA = clarification, PPT = precipitation, PUR = purification by ultracentrifugation) produce a solution in which the glycoprotein level represents 66.7% of the total proteins. In the residue of capsids (CAP), these glycoproteins do not represent more than 1%.

Adjuvant: The addition of an adjuvant to these viral subunit antigens is essential in order to assure satisfactory immunogenicity. Improvements in oil emulsion technology have lead to a better safety-adjuvanticity compromise. For this vaccine, the adjuvant concerned is a fluid oil-in-water type emulsion, below 18°C. The base of the emulsion is paraffin oil. The emulsion is perfectly safe when used via the deep intramuscular route in pigs (recommended injection route for this species). But it is also safe via the subcutaneous route which is the recommended injection route for cats and dogs.

QUALITY CONTROL METHODS FOR THE SUBUNIT VACCINE

Quality control methods used for the vaccine are in total conformity with the requirements of the European Pharmacopeia which are common to all vaccines and thus will not be presented in this chapter. It is, however, interesting to present the results of the intrinsic potency assays performed in pigs with industrial batches of vaccine, either with the Kojnok strain (non deleted) or with the KaH strain (deleted).

Direct testing in pigs - technique

The potency assay evaluates the immunogenicity of Geskypur in pigs by virulent challenge. The immune status is measured by recording the weight gain. The vaccine is administered according to the recommended method of use: vaccination of 5 susceptible pigs (weighing about 25 kg) with 1 dose (2 ml) of a batch of vaccine, via the deep intramuscular route in the neck region. The pigs are observed for 21 days. At the end of this period, the 5 vaccinated pigs and the 5 control pigs are weighed individually and challenged by instillation, into each nostril, of 1 ml (10^8 CCID50) of virulent virus, strain NIA-3. The pigs are then observed for 7 days and are weighed individually at the end of this period. Any dead pigs are also weighed. The criterion of protection is based on mortality and on an index (ΔG7), which is the difference between the relative mean daily weight gain of the vaccinated pigs and of the control pigs 7 days after challenge. A minimum discriminating value of 1 for the ΔG7 index has been calculated after the mathematic analysis of results from 41 batches of vaccine and about 500 pigs (Stellmann *et al.*, 1988). This value is significant for distinguishing vaccinated pigs from control pigs.

Examples and potency results in pigs

Selection of the amount of antigen per dose: Vaccines were prepared with variable amounts of glycoprotein antigen, the volume of the dose and the adjuvant remaining constant. The vaccines were tested using the ΔG7 vaccination-challenge technique. The amount of antigen per dose was selected as being 10μg, the best quality-price compromise (Table 3).

TABLE 3 Selection of the amount of antigen per dose

	2 μg	10μg	50μg
Non-deleted vaccine	1.38*	2.37	3.51
	1.71	2.26	2.16
Deleted vaccine	2.19	2.14	3.09
	1.18	1.81	1.91

* ΔG7 in pigs

Results of comparative potency of 6 batches of non-deleted vaccine and 6 batches of deleted vaccine: Six successive batches of industrial vaccine prepared using the Kojnok strain (non-deleted) gave the following results in ΔG7: 1.8 - 1.8 - 2.6 - 2.3 - 2.37 and 3.05 (m = 2.32). Six other successive batches of industrial vaccine, prepared using the KaH strain (deleted) gave the following results in ΔG7: 2.2 - 1.8 - 1.76 - 1.98 - 2.8 and 2.78 (m = 2.22).

Table 4 shows detailed results of 2 batches of vaccines (Brun *et al.*, 1988).

TABLE 4 Comparison of potency in pigs of 2 batches of subunit vaccine

Modalities		Weight (in kg) challenge day	on day 7 post challenge	M.R.D.G.*	
Deleted vaccine:					
controls	n.	29.6	24	- 2.82	
	s.d.	2.52	2.55	0.71	ΔG7 = 2.80
vaccinates	n.	28.30	28.10	0.02	
	s.d.	3.25	3.4	1.10	
Non-deleted vaccine:					
controls	n.	36.6	32.70	- 1.90	
	s.d.	8.91	9.30	1.43	ΔG7 = 3.05
vaccinates	n.	27.80	29.90	1.15	
	s.d.	3.25	2.54	0.76	

* M.R.D.G. = Mean Relative Daily Weight Gain

Results of comparative potency tests in piglets with passive immunity: Piglets born from sows vaccinated twice during gestation at about 6 weeks and 3 weeks prior to farrowing, were challenged as well as control piglets, at the age of 7 or 15 days with 1000 LD_{50} of the Kojnok challenge strain (0.5 ml into each nostril).

Table 5 summarizes the results of the maternal immunity obtained with either the deleted vaccine or the non-deleted vaccine.

TABLE 5 Maternal immunity in piglets obtained with deleted and non-deleted vaccines

	Mean VN antibody titer (log 10) of sows post farrowing		Protection of piglets at 7 and 15 days of age	
Deleted vaccine	1.95	6 sows	22/24	controls: 1/18
Non-deleted vaccine	2.00	31 sows	124/136	controls: 0/62

Neutralization test

The standardized technique in cell culture with constant virus and variable sera was applied to all the vaccinated and control pigs on the day of challenge. The analysis of the results demonstrates that the virus-neutralizing (VN) antibody titers, although effective serological controls of vaccination, cannot be retained as a protection criterion against virulent challenge.

Potency test in cats and dogs

Four groups of dogs (a total of 46 dogs) and 4 groups of cats (a total of 30 cats) were vaccinated with 1 dose (1 ml) via the subcutaneous route with Geskypur. Boosters were given 14 to 21 days later and certain dogs were given a third vaccinal injection 67 days after the first. Series of virulent challenges were carried out in vaccinated and control cats and dogs, after varying periods of immunity and up to 6 months following primary vaccination. All animals were kept for 1 month after virulent challenge. Serum samples were taken throughout the entire trial period for Aujeszky's disease antibody titration. All the control dogs (12/12) and cats (8/8) which received the challenge dose of 10^7 CCID50 via the oronasal route died within 5 to 11 days following the administration of the Kojnok challenge strain. Thirty one of the 34 vaccinated dogs were protected. The 3 vaccinated dogs which were not protected had received 2 injections. However, all cats vaccinated with 2 injections were protected from the virulent challenge up to 90 days following primary vaccination. An increase in specific antibody was observed in all vaccinated animals, but no correlation was found between VN antibodies and protection.

SUBUNIT VACCINES (NON-DELETED OR DELETED) AS A WAY TO DIFFERENTIATE BETWEEN VACCINATED AND CONVALESCENT ANIMALS

The exclusive use of inactivated viral structural antigens could help to differentiate between convalescent pigs or pigs vaccinated with certain modified live vaccine strains and pigs vaccinated with Geskypur. All that would need to be done is to test the reactivity of the sera against the non-structural gX protein.

In the case of subunit vaccines, the absence of viral capsid proteins, lead us to analyse the reactivity of the sera of pigs recovering from a virulent challenge, or immunized with several injections of Geskypur vaccine. This analysis was done using the Western blotting system: electrophoresis of the purified virus treated with detergent and betamercaptoethanol, transfer onto nitrocellulose, contact with 1/100 diluted sera and revelation by peroxidase conjugated antibodies. Reactivities are visible in Fig. 4. The evaluation of the reactions is done by photometric reading and results can be found in Fig. 5. The kinetics of appearance of gII and gIII specific antibodies are very different in convalescent pigs and infected pigs. The antibodies to the p 42 capsid protein are observed in convalescent pigs, and, unfortunately

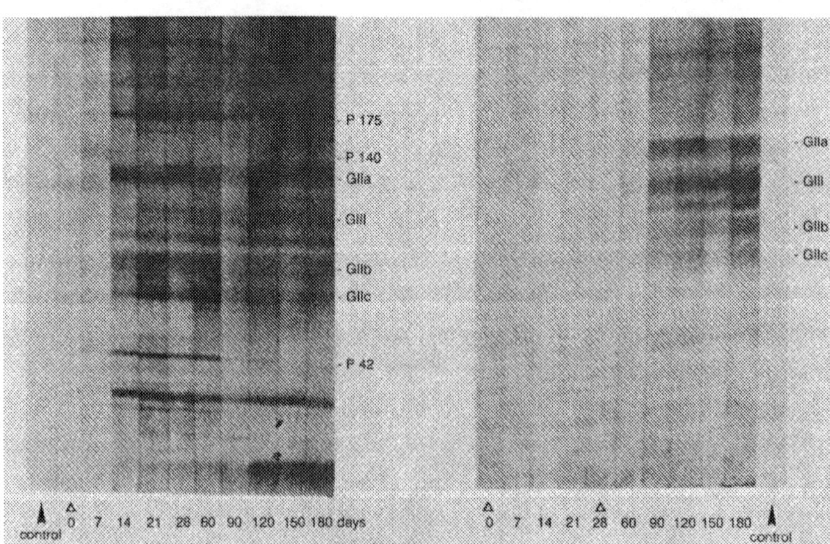

Fig. 4 **Affinity immunoblot analysis of sera from infected and vaccinated pigs.**

only at significant levels between 7 and 60 days post infection. This is a means of distinguishing between convalescent pigs (and possibly pigs immunized with live vaccines) and pigs vaccinated with Geskypur. However, this method is too complicated to apply in routine use. The search for other techniques (Van Oirschot *et al.*, 1986), the use of strains deleted in the proteins which are not essential for the appearance of immunity, and the preparation of Geskypur with the KaH strain deleted in gI and gp63 (Mettenleiter *et al.*, 1987) offer a significant opportunity to distinguish between vaccinated and infected animals in the field.

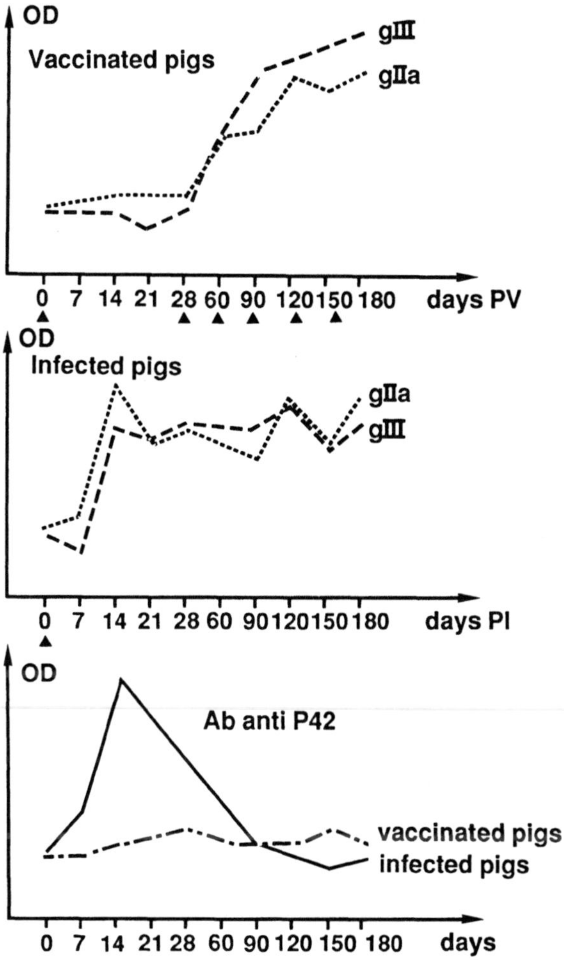

Fig. 5 Kinetics of antibodies against viral fractions. Arrows indicate days of inoculation.

REFERENCES

Brun, A., Vandeputte, J., Chappuis, G. and Fargeaud, D. 1988. Comparative study of the activity of 2 subunit vaccines against Aujeszky's disease: deleted and non-deleted. IPVS Congress, Rio de Janeiro, Brazil, August 14-17th.

Chappuis, G., Benoit-Jeannin, C. and Fargeaud, D. 1981. Rhinotracheite feline: vaccin inactivé purifié et modèle expérimental. 17th Int. Congress on Herpesvirus - Standardization of Immunological procedures, Lyon, France. Develop. biol. Standard, **52,** 485-491 (S. Karger, Basel, 1982).

Fargeaud, D., Benoit-Jeannin, C., Kato, F. and Chappuis, G. 1984. Biochemical study of the Feling Herpesvirus 1: Identification of glycoprotein by affinity. Arch. Virol., **80,** 69-82.

Hampl, H., Ben-Porat, T., Ehrlicher, L., Habermehl, K.O. and Kaplan, A.S. 1984. Characterization of the envelope proteins of pseudorabies virus. J. Virol., **52,** 583-590.

Mettenleiter, T.C., Scheurs, C., Zuckermann, F. and Ben-Porat, T. 1987. Role of Pseudorabies virus glycoprotein gI in virus release from infected cells. J. Virol., **61,** 2764-2769.

Stellmann, C., Vannier, P., Chappuis, G., Brun, A., Dauvergne, M., Fargeaud, D., Bugand, M. and Colson, X. 1988. Pseudorabies vaccines, vaccine potency testing in pigs. Proposal of a quantitative criterion and a minimum requirement. J. Biol. Stand., **17,** in press.

Van Oirschot, J.T., Rziha, H.J., Moonen, P.J.L.M., Pol, J.M.A. and Van Zaane, D. 1986. Differentiation of serum antibodies from pigs vaccinated or infected with Aujeszky's disease virus by a competitive enzyme immunoassay. J. Gen. Virol., **67,** 1179-1182.

LATENCY CHARACTERISTICS OF PSEUDORABIES VACCINE VIRUSES

H.J. Rziha, V. Ohlinger*, D. Lütticken**, N. Visser***

*Federal Research Centre For Animal Virus Diseases,
D-7400 Tübingen, FRG
**Intervet Int. B.V., NL 5830 AA Boxmeer, The Netherlands

ABSTRACT

First results of a study initiated to investigate the latency characteristics of pseudorabies virus (PRV) vaccine strains and mutants are presented. By DNA hybridization it could be shown that a gI⁻/TK⁻ PRV construct (strain Begonia) replicated only marginally in different neural tissues and tonsils of swine early after application. Four months later neither infectious virus nor viral DNA was detectable in the immunosuppressed animals. In contrast, swine immunosuppressed 4 months after vaccination with the gI^-/TK^+ strain NIA-4 exhibited viral DNA in various organs, but virus was not recoverable. Furthermore, superinfection of pigs with virulent PRV 2 months after NIA-4 vaccination showed the establishment of a reactivable, latent wild-type virus infection.

INTRODUCTION

Pseudorabies virus (PRV) establishes a latent infection in various neural tissues of swine (Rziha *et al.*, 1986), and virus can be reactivated by immunosuppressive treatment (Mock *et al.*, 1980; Wittmann *et al.*, 1983; Thawley *et al.*, 1984; Van Oirschot and Gielkens, 1984). The persistence of PRV in extraneural tissues is indicated by the presence of viral DNA (Rziha *et al.*, in preparation), although the actual role of those cells in the establishment, maintenance and reactivation of latency remains to be elucidated. For the use of PRV live vaccines it is important to know whether vaccine virus might become latent and be reactivated. Furthermore, the ability of a live vaccine to influence the establishment of a latent field virus infection in vaccinated swine is rather unclear. To investigate these questions (1) swine vaccinated with the attenuated NIA-4 strain or with a glycoprotein I-negative (gI^-)/thymidine kinase-negative (TK^-) constructed vaccine and (2) vaccinated pigs after superinfection with wild-type PRV were tested for virus excretion, virus recovery and for the presence of viral DNA in numerous organ tissues. These are the first experiments of a study including different constructed deletion mutants of PRV to

J. T. van Oirschot (ed.), Vaccination and Control of Aujeszky's Disease, 79–85.

investigate also the possible role of viral gene functions in latency and reactivation.

MATERIALS AND METHODS

Experimental design

A. Two to 6-day-old swine were inoculated intranasally (IN) and intramuscularly (IM) with 10^6 $TCID_{50}$ of a gI⁻/TK⁻ constructed PRV strain designated Begonia. The gI gene was removed from the genome of PRV strain NIA-3 as described (Quint *et al.*, 1987). One group of animals was killed at 6 days after infection (p.i.), different organ tissues were removed, snap frozen and tested for the presence of viral DNA. At 6 weeks after inoculation with 10^8 $TCID_{50}$ Begonia another group of 6 animals was treated with prednisolone (15 mg/kg of body weight) for 4 consecutive days, killed 4 weeks later and different organ tissues were removed.

B. Groups of 4 pigs (8-week-old) were inoculated IN (10^6 $TCID_{50}$) with the virulent strain Phylaxia (groups B.1 and B.2) or with the attenuated, gI⁻ strain NIA-4 (groups B.3 and B.4). Two months p.i. animals recovered from primary infection were superinfected with the NIA-4 strain (group B.1) or with the Phylaxia strain (group B.3) and after an additional 2 months the pigs were immunosuppressed for reactivation of latent PRV. The animals of groups B.2 and B.4 remained for 4 months before immunosuppression. Various organ tissues of all animals were tested for virus recovery and for the presence of viral DNA.

Virus recovery was achieved by co-cultivation on permissive culture cells (Rziha *et al.*, 1986). In addition, direct virus titration assays of homogenized organs were performed.

Total DNA was phenol-extracted from the organ tissues and viral DNA was detected by Southern blot and dot or slot blot hybridization using in vitro ^{32}P-labelled cloned PRV DNA-fragments as probes (Rziha *et al.*, 1986).

RESULTS AND DISCUSSION

Experiment A

Although the pigs vaccinated with the Begonia strain excreted virus at day 4 and 5 p.i., only very low amounts of viral DNA could be detected in the different neural tissues and in the tonsils at 6 days p.i. After slot blot hybridization a semiquantitative determination of the PRV DNA concentration present could be made. As shown in Fig. 1, none of the organ tissues tested contained more than 1.0 to 2.0 PRV genome copies per cell. Usually, during the acute phase of wild-type virus (e.g. Phylaxia) infection between 10 to 100 genome copies per cell are found in these organs (Rziha *et al.*, 1986). The specificity of the results of the slot blot hybridization was proved by Southern blotting of the restriction enzyme-cleaved organ DNA (not shown). All positive specimens showed the presence of the shortened Bam HI fragment 7 due to the gI deletion. These data indicate that at least in the central (CNS) and the peripheral nervous system (PNS) as well as in the tonsils a markedly reduced replication of the gI⁻/TK⁻ mutant virus had occurred.

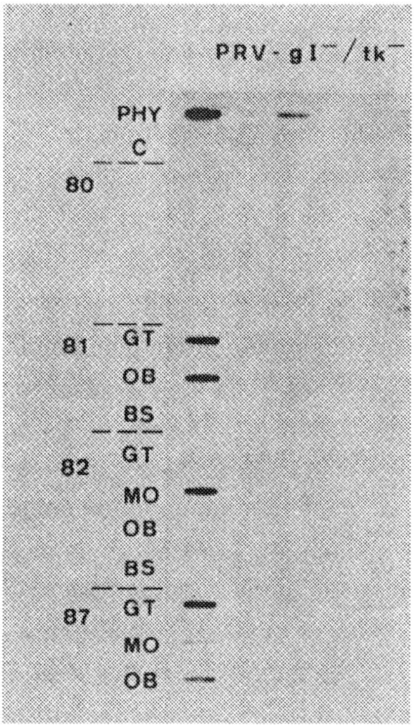

Fig. 1 Presence of Begonia DNA in neural tissues (for abbreviations see text) of 4 pigs (Nos. 80, 81, 82 and 87) at 6 days p.i. Extracted organ DNA was slotted onto nitrocellulose filter (1.slot 10 μg, 3.slot 2 μg) and hybridized with ^{32}P-nick translated cloned Bam HI fragment 7. Lane PHY represents reconstruction control: 0.2 μg virion DNA and 10 μg uninfected GT DNA were slotted undiluted (1.slot), diluted 1:10 (2.slot) and 1:100 (3.slot). In lane C 10 μg uninfected GT DNA only were transferred.

The immunosuppressive treatment of the pigs, 6 weeks after vaccination with 10^8TCID$_{50}$ (a very high dose of virus), did not result in rescue of infectious virus from the brain stem, lymph nodes, tonsils, and lungs. After DNA hybridization viral genome could not be detected in the brain stem, medulla oblongata, olfactory bulb or trigeminal ganglia of all 6 animals. As proved by reconstruction experiments the limit of sensitivity in these hybridization assays was less than 0.1 PRV genome copies per cell. Thus, one can suggest that no or only very low amounts of gI⁻/TK⁻

virus persisted in those tissues, which corroborates the failure of virus recovery by co-cultivation experiments.

Apparently, during the acute state of infection the Begonia strain replicated only to a low extent and consequently no latent infection might have been established. However, one cannot exclude that undetectable, low amounts of latent mutant virus can persist, which are not easily reactivable.

Experiment B

This experiment was designed to examine (1) whether the gI$^-$, attenuated strain NIA-4 can establish a reactivable, latent infection; (2) whether wild-type virus superinfection of NIA-4-vaccinated pigs will result in reactivable latency of Phylaxia virus; (3) which virus strain can be reactivated after superinfection of either NIA-4 or Phylaxia-infected swine.

(1) After application of NIA-4 (group B.3 and B.4) only 1 of the 8 pigs excreted the virus at 5 days p.i. During the reactivation of these pigs (group B.4), 4 months later no virus excretion occurred as tested with nasal swabs taken daily. In addition, virus could not be recovered from various neural and extraneural tissues. Virusspecific DNA, however, could be detected in varying concentrations in a wide range of organ tissues and cells. This is demonstrated representatively for 1 animal of group B.4 in Fig. 2. Less than 0.3 genome copies per cell were present in the retropharyngeal lymph nodes (RLN), lungs (LU), tonsils (TO), thymus (THY), macrophages (Mø), spleen (SP), trigeminal ganglia (GT), and brain stem (BS). In the medulla oblongata (MO), the olfactory bulb (BO) and in the nasal mucosa (NM) between 2 to 5 genome copies per cell were detectable. In spite of the presence of viral DNA, no infectious virus could be rescued from these animals. The reason for this discrepancy remains to be elucidated. One might speculate that the gI$^-$/TK$^+$ strain NIA-4 possesses a reduced ability to reactivate, albeit this virus seems to invade and to persist not only in the PNS and CNS. However, it has to be proven that the protocol of reactivation, which is well adapted to the virulent strain Phylaxia, can be also successfully used for other PRV strains or mutants.

(2) Four animals (group B.3) were superinfected with strain Phylaxia 2 months after vaccination with NIA-4. Two pigs excreted virus during the immunosuppressive treatment. Similarly as in group B.4, viral DNA was demonstrable in all organs tested, except of trigeminal ganglia (Fig. 2), which was also the case in group B.1 (infection with Phylaxia preceded NIA-4 infection). These results principally correspond to those obtained after reactivation of animals only infected with strain Phylaxia. The significance of the different PRV DNA concentrations in the different organ cells,

particularly the absence of the viral genome in the trigeminal ganglia of the superinfected pigs, is questionable; more thorough investigations with greater number of animals must be awaited. None of the animals of groups B.3 and B.1 shed virus.

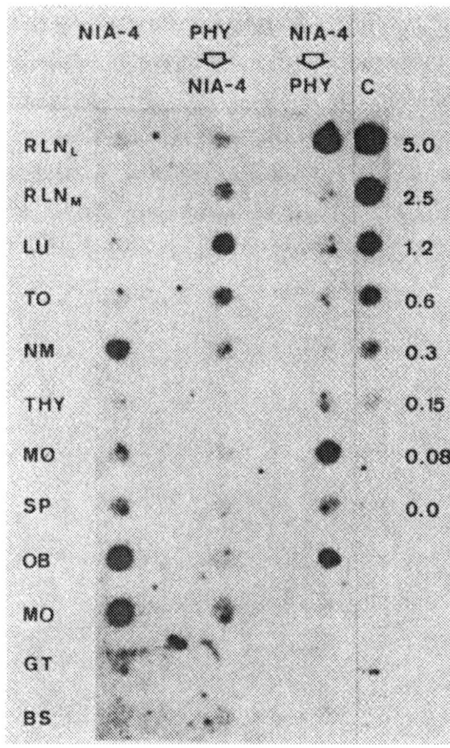

Fig. 2 Detection of viral DNA in various organ tissues (horizontal rows; for abbreviations see text) of immunosuppressed animals infected with the indicated virus combinations (vertical rows; row 1 = group B.4, row 2 - group B.1, row 3 = group B.3). Row C represents a reconstruction control of 10 μg uninfected lung cell DNA containing the amounts of PRV genome copies per cell as indicated on the right. Each dot contains 10 μg DNA; annealing as in Fig. 1.

These results already indicate that vaccination with strain NIA-4 apparently could not protect the animals against the induction of a reactivable, latent infection of virulent PRV. In fact, restriction enzyme analysis of the excreted virus of group B.3 animals revealed the occurrence of the superinfecting strain Phylaxia. This can be seen in Fig. 3 showing the results of Southern blot hybridization using the radiolabelled cloned Bam HI fragment 7 or total virion DNA (not shown) as probes. In all cases only the wild-type virusspecific fragment 7 was detected.

In summary, the following conclusions can be drawn. (1) The gI^-/TK^- PRV construct had invaded the PNS, CNS, and the tonsils, but replication seemed to occur at very low levels and neither reactivable, latent virus nor latent viral DNA was detectable. These results support earlier indications that TK$^-$ PRV strains might have a reduced potential of establishing latent infections (Tenser *et al.*, 1983; Lomniczi *et al.*, 1984; Kit *et al.*, 1985). In contrast, the genome of the gI$^-$/TK$^+$ strain NIA-4 was detected in various organs of immunosuppressed pigs (6 weeks p.i.), but infectious virus could be not recovered. To what an extent gI might be involved in the reactivation of latent PRV remains to be seen. Our results indicate that reactivation of strain NIA-4 is more difficult to achieve than reactivation of the Phylaxia strain. (2) Vaccination of swine with strain NIA-4 did not protect the animals against a reactivable, latent infection of virulent challenge PRV.

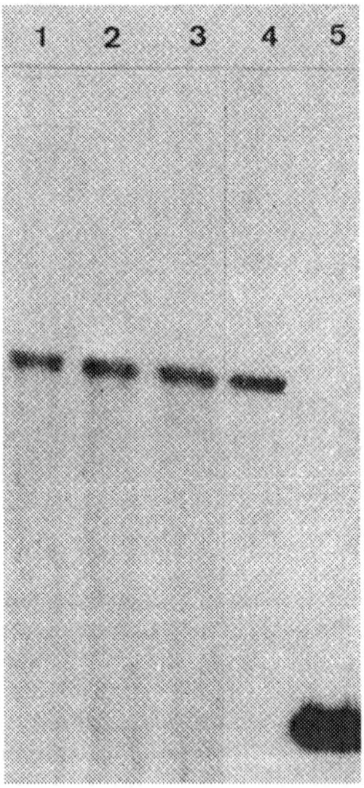

Fig.3 Southern blot hybridization of Bam HI-cleaved DNA obtained from excreted virus (nasal swabs) of immunosuppressed animals 4 months after infection with (1) Phylaxia, (2) Phylaxia and NIA-4 superinfection, and (3) NIA-4 and Phylaxia superinfection. Cleaved virion DNA of strain Phylaxia (lane 4) and strain NIA-4 (lane 5) was included; annealing as in Fig. 1.

REFERENCES

Kit, S., Kit, M. and Pirtle, E.C. 1985. Attenuated properties of thymidine kinase-negative deletion mutant of pseudorabies virus. Am. J. Vet. Res., **46,** 1359-1367.

Lomniczi, B., Watanabe, S., Ben-Porat, T. and Kaplan, A.S. 1984. Genetic basis of the neurovirulence of pseudorabies virus. J. Virol., **52,** 198-205.

Mock, R.E., Crandell, R.A. and Mesfin, G.M. 1980. Induced latency in pseudorabies virus vaccinated pigs. Can. J. Comp. Med., **45,** 56-59.

Quint, W., Gielkens, A.L.J., Van Oirschot, J.T., Berns, A.J.M. and Cuypers, H.T. 1987. Construction and characterization of deletion mutants of pseudorabies virus: A new generation of live vaccines. J. Gen. Virol., **68,** 523-534.

Rziha, H.J., Mettenleiter, T.C., Ohlinger, V.F. and Wittmann, G. 1986. Herpesvirus (pseudorabies virus) latency in swine: Occurrence and physical state of viral DNA in neural tissues. Virol., **155,** 600-613.

Tenser, R.B., Ressel, S.J., Fralish, F.A. and Jones, J.C. 1983. The role of pseudorabies virus thymidine kinase expression in trigeminal ganglion infection. J. Gen. Virol., **64,** 1369-1373.

Thawley, D.G., Solorzano, R.F. and Johnson, M.E. 1984. Confirmation of pseudorabies virus infection using virus recrudescence by dexamethasone treatment and in vitro lymphocyte stimulation. Am. J. Vet. Res., **45,** 981-983.

Van Oirschot, J.T. and Gielkens, A.L.J. 1984. In vivo and in vitro reactivation of latent pseudorabies virus in pigs born to vaccinated sows. Am. J. Vet. Res., **45,** 567-571.

Wittmann, G., Ohlinger, V.F. and Rziha, H.J. 1983. Occurrence and reactivation of latent Aujeszky's disease virus following challenge in previously vaccinated pigs. Arch. Virol., **75,** 29-41.

RISK ASSESSMENT OF FIELD RELEASE OF ENGINEERED AUJESZKY'S DISEASE VIRUS VACCINES: PRINCIPLES OF APPROACH

A. Jestin, P. Vannier

Ministère de l'Agriculture, Direction Générale de l'Alimentation,
Station de Pathologie Porcine, B.P. 9, 22440 Ploufragan, France

ABSTRACT

The advent of recombinant DNA techniques has made possible the manipulation of natural DNA sequences within an organism in order to change functions of the organism. Different Aujeszky's disease virus vaccines have been produced by these recombinant techniques. Some of them have been submitted to French agriculture authorities for registration as live viral vaccine for pigs. The question of the risk of deliberate field release of such engineered viruses has been arisen. The most problematic modifications at the molecular level are identified and are discussed in theory: modification of the DNA sequence, alteration of the biological properties of the encoded protein. These engineered live vaccines may be released if no problematic modifications are identified and if the vaccinal virus does not spread from the vaccinated pigs.

INTRODUCTION

The application of recombinant DNA techniques to Aujeszky's disease (AD) virus (ADV) has a relatively recent history. The first modification attempt to lower the pathogenicity of the virus was the inactivation of the thymidine kinase gene; it rendered ADV nonpathogenic (Kit *et al.*, 1985). The second modification was the induction of deletions in structural or nonstructural proteins for the purpose of creating a diagnostic marker. Deliberate release of these engineered organisms used as live viral vaccines for pigs, arises the question of the risk of such modified viruses for pigs and of their possible dissemination in nature. However, conventionally modified live virus vaccines have been widely used and found to be safe to control AD.

At present it is possible to speculate about the new properties of the modified ADV vaccines in relation with insertion of a foreign DNA or a deletion within the genome which encodes for a new or a modified protein, or destroys a protein, respectively. Our objective is to evaluate theoretically the consequences of the

J. T. van Oirschot (ed.), Vaccination and Control of Aujeszky's Disease, 87–92.

possible field release of the genetically engineered ADV vaccines.

IDENTIFICATION OF MOST PROBLEMATIC MODIFICATIONS AND MOLECULAR BASIS OF SAFETY MEASURES

Modification of the DNA sequence

1. Deletion of a gene.

The new phenotype is the result of a deletion of some nucleotides of the protein coding sequence. To reconstruct a functional gene, the sequence with the same or nearly the same coding possibilities as the deleted nucleotides would have to be recreated. There is no known mechanism for spontaneous generation of a given sequence of this size, such as exists for the spontaneous reversion of a point mutation or single base deletion. In all cases the sequence of the fragment before and after the deletion has to be determined. The minimum size of the deleted fragment is not easy to precise. A deletion of 200 nucleotides in an enzymatic protein gene usually is enough to destroy its biological properties. In other cases a major part of the gene has to be deleted to destroy the function of the coded protein. In all cases large deletions are easily detected in electrophoretic patterns of restriction fragments and are used as markers.

Different computer analysis programs, based on published research papers, either for proteins or nucleic acids, can be used to compare the homology between sequences coding for 2 proteins with similar biological properties.

When the genome of a vaccine strain carries 2 deletions, for instance the first in a gene coding for virulence and the second one in a nonessential gene, for use as a "serological marker", the probability of creating a new virus (recombination) with a mixture of this vaccine strain and a wild-type strain has to be considered. The probability of creating a virulent ADV strain with a deletion in the serological marker protein and an avirulent strain without the serological marker is theoretically present. The probability of recombination in that way is dependent, among other things, on the genomic distance between the 2 genes coding for the proteins.

2. Insertion of a foreign DNA fragment.

The problematic aspect of the presence of foreign DNA inserted in the ADV genome is the ability of a naturally occurring recombination event between the modified ADV genome and other organisms with the inserted DNA sequences.

2.1. Transient presence of a foreign DNA insert. When during the construction procedure of a deletion mutant, foreign DNA has transiently been present in the viral genome, it is necessary to confirm that these foreign DNA sequences are not present in the deleted vaccine virus strain. Two approaches can be used for this purpose: sequencing of the gene that carries the deletion, or the use of DNA probes in Southern blotting. In that case the probe contains the entire fragment of the transiently inserted foreign DNA.

2.2. Persistence of a foreign DNA insert. Viral, bacterial (plasmidal, chromosomal) DNA sequences are present in the ADV genome. Although it is highly unlikely that recombination events occur, answers to the following questions are not known. Can this insert DNA be used as a vehicle to introduce foreign DNA in the ADV genome? Can the ADV genome serve as a source of foreign DNA for other viruses or bacteria by means of its inserted DNA? Are the engineered vaccines a vehicle for the escape of ADV genes? When the vaccinal virus is accidentally disseminated in the piggery, can the procaryotic DNA fragment inserted in the vaccine virus strain facilitate the entry in a bacterium and thereby introduce ADV genes into bacterial DNA?

2.3. Identification of genomic markers for the precise detection of the released organism. Electrophoretic patterns of digested genomic DNA are useful to compare different ADV strains; engineered vaccine viruses can be easily identified in that way. However, if, in some cases, the DNA insertion destroys one endonuclease restriction site, the studied fragment may be located in the upper part of the gel and can be detected by DNA probes using Southern blot procedures. Such techniques have to be detailed by the producers of these engineered ADV vaccines, in terms of rapidity of use and specificity.

2.4. Study of genetic stability of recombinant ADV vaccines. After passage of the vaccine virus strain in pigs, the strain is recovered and studied by DNA restriction enzyme analysis. The DNA electrophoretic pattern must be stable and by DNA probes, in Southern blots, the presence of inserted foreign DNA has to be confirmed. At least 5 passages in swine have to be made to be sure the virus strain is genetically stable.

Alterations of the biological properties of the virus induced by the encoded protein.

1. Expression of a new protein in ADV.

Introduction in the ADV genome of foreign DNA encoding for a protein can confer new properties to the engineered vaccine. When, for instance, the ADV genome is recombined with a fragment from another mammalian herpesvirus it can acquire a functional gene which plays a role in determining species susceptibility. Consequently, other animal species may become susceptible for such an engineered ADV vaccine strain. Therefore, the susceptibility of other mammalian animals for the engineered vaccine could be an important item in the discussion on the release of engineered ADV vaccines.

2. Expression of a truncated protein.

The introduction of deletions in an open reading frame results in modification of the primary, secondary and/or tertairy structures of the encoded protein. The chemical alteration will inactivate or modify the biological activity of that protein. Such modifications may confer new tissue tropism or other new properties to the vaccine virus.

BARRIERS TO VIRAL GENE RELEASE INTO THE ENVIRONMENT

The putative transfer of recombinant viral DNA molecules from the vaccinated organisms to other populations in the environment may be an important factor in assessing the risks of deliberate release of genetically engineered organisms into this environment. Two types of barriers may theoretically reduce the putative transfer from the vaccinated organisms into an ecosystem.

"Genes mixing barrier" limiting the free transfer of vaccine strain DNA.

The nature of gene exchange in recombination events between 2 viruses requires simultaneous entry of the viral genomes into the same cell. In natural cases of AD in unvaccinated swine, the virus is mostly found in the regional lymph nodes draining the nasopharynx, in the central nervous system, in trachea and lungs. In vaccinated swine, the probability of recombination between the genomes of an engineered vaccine and a field strain is extremely low, when the vaccine is injected intramuscularly in the neck and when the multiplication of the vaccine virus is restricted around the site of inoculation. Studies on dissemination of the vaccine virus in the pig have to be conducted to estimate for each vaccine the frequency of potential recombination with field virus. The absence of dissemination of the engineered vaccine virus in the organism is an important biological property.

There is a probability of recombination, although theoretically, when, accidently, 2 vaccines carrying different deletions are mixed and injected by the same syringe. Recently, it has been established that a mixture of 2 avirulent herpes simplex virus strains when inoculated at the same site produced disease in mice due to complementation or recombination (Javier *et al.*, 1986).

"Genes exit barrier" limiting the free transfer of DNA between swine and the environment or other species

1. Direct spread by airborne transmission.

The first step of possible gene exchanges is transmission of the vaccine virus from vaccinated to unvaccinated pigs or other animal species. Studies indicated that airborne transmission of wild-type ADV occurs among swine and from swine to cattle. Studies have to be performed to prove that protein modification does not modify or enhance tropism of the vaccine virus for the lung and as a result does not increase viral dissemination in this way. Recently, a new porcine coronavirus, the TGE-like coronavirus, spread over Europe by airborne transmission. Molecular studies showed that ultrastructural modifications are probably limited to some parts of the peplomeric proteins (Laude *et al.*, 1988).

2. Indirect release into the environment.

Various wild animals have been experimentally infected with field strains of ADV. These experiments demonstrated that these wild animals cannot considered to be virus reservoirs. Experiments have to be done to determine whether carnivores (fox, dog, cat) that have eaten some muscular parts of a previously vaccinated pig, will shed the engineered vaccine virus.

STANDARDIZATION OF MODEL AND LIMITED FIELD TRIAL EXPERIMENTS

Most widely used live virus vaccines have been evaluated under experimental conditions before studying them under field conditions, even on a small scale. To assess the risk related to the use of engineered vaccines, trials under experimental conditions have to be done to predict the biology of the modified organisms. As a second step, pigs on a few farms can be vaccinated. These herds have to be located in an uninfected region. Finally, as a third step a similar experiment has to be conducted in an infected region.

CONCLUSION

This article tries to consider the question of risk assessment of releasing recombinant DNA engineered ADV vaccines into the environment. At present, decisions to release such an organism are based on the examination of the molecular construction and on the biological properties of the vaccine virus ("gene mixing and gene exit"). The most problematic modifications at the molecular level, as well as the potential properties, of the engineered vaccines are identified and discussed. It is clear that the hazards associated with the environmental release of recombinant DNA engineered organisms cannot be evaluated in theory. At present, engineered ADV vaccines can be released when a multidisciplinary commission does not identify problematic modifications at the molecular level.

REFERENCES

Javier, R.T., Sedarati, F. and Stevens, J.G. 1986. Two avirulent herpes simplex viruses viruses generate lethal recombinants in vivo. Science, **234,** 746-748.

Kit, S., Kit, M. and Pirtle, E.C. 1985. Attenuated properties of thymidine kinase-negative deletion mutant of pseudorabies virus. Am. J. Vet. Res., **46,** 1359-1367.

Laude, H., Gelfi, J., Rasschaert, D. and Delmas, B., 1988. Caracterisation antigenique du coronavirus respiratoire porcine à l'aide d'anticorps monoclonaux dirigés contre le virus de la gastro-entérite transmissible. J. Rech. Porc., **20,** 89-94.

MOLECULAR EPIDEMIOLOGY OF AUJESZKY'S DISEASE IN HUNGARY

B. Lomniczi, E. Nagy, A. Kükedi, L. Zsák*

Veterinary Medical Research Institute
of the Hungarian Academy of Sciences
1581 Budapest, Pf. 18, Hungary
*Department of Veterinary Microbiology and Immunology
University of Guelph
Guelph, Ontario N1G 2W1, Canada

ABSTRACT

The DNAs of 560 field isolates of Aujeszky's disease virus (ADV) were analyzed by restriction enzymes Bam HI and Kpn I. These strains were isolated between 1975 and 1988; 509 were derived from 290 pig farms, while 51 were isolated from pets (dogs and cats). Based on DNA cleavage site variations, ADV strains isolated in Hungary could be classified into 10 groups. The majority of the strains belong to the prototype variety represented by strain PRV-Ka (Rixon and Ben-Porat, 1979). This group can be subdivided on the basis of the mobility of Bam fragment 5' and this marker remained stable for years on the same farm. The prototype variety colonizes 80% of the pig farms, while strains with 9 different cleavage site markers were found in 20% of the herds. Strains with the second most frequent marker (Kpn F_1+F_2) colonize 11% of the farms and have become the dominant ones in one county reflecting the commercial activity of a single pig-breeder. With the help of DNA markers and local evidence on the circumstances of new AD outbreaks epidemiological investigations were carried out to shed light on the origin and/or the mode of introduction of ADV infection in particular cases.

INTRODUCTION

Molecular biology has provided some useful tools that allow further differentiation of virus groups where conventional virological methods have stopped. These include fingerprinting of virus nucleic acids and proteins. Mutations in viral genomes constantly elicit large numbers of structural varieties. Some of these varieties may be selected for in a group of host animals, thus generating virus diversity in the field. Therefore one would expect that virus strains isolated from unrelated disease outbreaks may not be identical, while epidemiologically related cases yield indistinguishable strains. If we have tools sensitive enough to reveal structural differences between virus strains isolated from unrelated outbreaks, then

J. T. van Oirschot (ed.), Vaccination and Control of Aujeszky's Disease, 93–102.

one is able to trace the route of a particular strain through a succession of presumably epidemiologically related outbreaks. Restriction enzyme (RE) analysis of the DNA has been successfully used to differentiate between strains of various herpesviruses (Hayward *et al.*, 1975; Buchman *et al.*, 1980) and field isolates of Aujeszky's disease (AD) virus (ADV) (Geck *et al.*, 1982; Gielkens and Berns, 1982; Ludwig *et al.*, 1982; Paul *et al.*, 1982; Ben-Porat *et al.*, 1984a,b; Gielkens *et al.*, 1984, 1985; Herrmann *et al.*, 1984; Pirtle *et al.*, 1984; Pritchett *et al.*, 1984; Todd and McFerran, 1985; Nishimori *et al.*, 1987). In a systematic study in Hungary we have analyzed the DNAs of 560 strains isolated on 290 pig farms and from pets (dogs and cats) and we have found 9 cleavage site markers (on 20% of farms) besides the prototype pattern. In a number of cases we combined knowledge of DNA patterns with information on the probable spread of infection and have proved or excluded hypotheses concerning epidemiological relationships between AD outbreaks.

MATERIALS AND METHODS

Permanent pig kidney (PK-15) cells were used to propagate virus strains.

ADV strains were kindly provided by the Veterinary Institutes in Hungary by the courtesy of Drs. Zsuzsa Máté, E. Mocsári, V. Palya and J. Tanyi.

Virus propagation, purification, DNA extraction and digestion with RE, agarose gel electrophoresis and Southern blot hybridization were done as described (Lomniczi *et al.*, 1984).

RESULTS

The DNAs of 509 ADV strains isolated on 290 pig farms in the last decade in Hungary were examined by REs Bam HI and Kpn I. In addition 51 strains were isolated from dogs and cats. The place and date of isolations were known as well as when repeated isolations were done on the same farm.

As reported (Gielkens *et al.*, 1985) differences between the DNA fragment patterns obtained by RE digestion and agarose gel electrophoresis are of 2 types: a) loss or gain of cleavage sites resulting in the emergence of new fragments due to fusion or cleavage; b) variation in the mobility of certain DNA fragments due to addition or deletion of sequences. ADV strains differing in the first type of changes will be called varieties of one another, while those of the second type will be called variants by analogy of the nomenclature applied to RNA virus strains with significant and slight differences of their oligonucleotide fingerprints, respectively (Clewley and Bishop, 1982).

Cleavage site differences

Fig. 1 shows RE patterns of the DNAs of ADV strains digested by Bam HI. Lane A is strain PRV-Ka (Rixon and Ben-Porat, 1979) that has been chosen as prototype. Lane B represents a strain whose fragment 3 has an extra Bam HI cleavage site, therefore it shows up as 2 subfragments (3a and 3b). This and the other cleavage site changes were confirmed by Southern hybridization (B. Lomniczi and T. Ben-Porat, unpublished data). Lane C shows the DNA pattern of a variety where 2 extra fragments appear above fragment 4, while fragment 10 and 12 are missing. These large fragments are the results of 2 different fusion events between fragments 5 and 10, and also between fragments 5 and 12. So these changes involve the loss of cleavage sites. The approximate molecular weights of the fusion fragments are somewhat smaller than the constituent fragments (Lomniczi *et al.*, 1984), indicating that the loss of cleavage sites was due to small deletions of approximately 0.2 dalton each. Lane D also reveals the appearance of 2 new fragments resulting from double fusion events: one between fragment 8' and 8, the other between fragment 8 and 13.

Figure 1

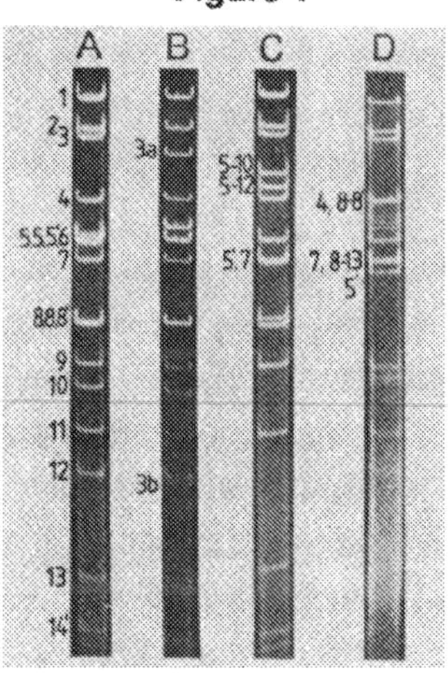

Figure 2

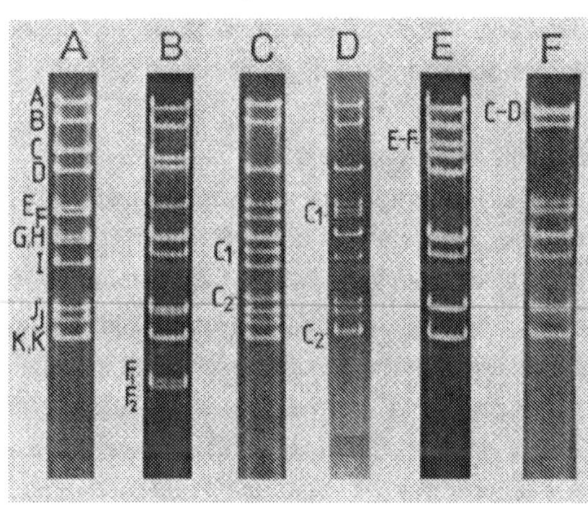

Electrophoretic patterns of DNA fragments of ADV strains obtained by digestion with RE Bam HI (fig. 1) and Kpn I (fig. 2). Lane A = prototype strain PRV-Ka (for others see text)

The existence of other DNA varieties was revealed by RE Kpn I, as shown on Fig. 2. Lane A represents the prototype pattern (strain PRV-Ka). Lane B is a variety where an extra Kpn I cleavage site appears on fragment F. Two additional cleavage sites appear in different location on fragment C (lanes C and D), and also on fragment B (not shown). Lanes E and F show varieties in which fragments E and F, and C and D are fused, respectively.

Variations in the mobility of DNA fragments

The majority of ADV strains isolated in Hungary belongs to the prototype variety. We have found, however, that the DNA patterns of ADV strains that colonize different pig farms are rarely identical. Differences between strains belonging to the prototype variety were often detected in the electrophoretic mobility of DNA fragments (a more detailed description will be published elsewhere). We have also found that fragments of variable size derive from the repeat regions or from the terminal part of the long unique sequences of the genome, as shown by others, too (Ben-Porat *et al.*, 1984a,b; Gielkens *et al.*, 1985). This, however, does not necessarily mean that strains should exhibit fragment variability when isolated repeatedly on the same farm. E.g. by analyzing several hundred strains it was noticed that Bam HI fragment 5' of most strains either comigrates with fragment 6 (Fig. 1, lanes A and B) or has a deletion of about 0.6 md and runs with fragment 7 (Fig. 1, lane C). It is interesting to note that strain AUJ that is regarded as an isolate made by A. Aujeszky (Paul *et al.*, 1982) and the PRV-Ka strain whose origin goes back to R.E. Shope, are very similar; their fragment 5' comigrates with fragment 6. Therefore, we, somewhat arbitrarily, regard these strain as an "old" type, whereas, those with a deletion on 5', are considered to be more recent variants.

Stability of DNA markers

If DNA markers are to be used for epidemiological investigation we must have proof of their stability under field conditions. This was obtained by showing that mobility of even the variable fragments did not change in strains isolated serially during the same outbreaks (Nagy, 1988) or only slightly in strains isolated on the same farm at intervals of several months (Nagy *et al.*, 1985a). Some DNA markers (e.g. Kpn $F_1 + F_2$, Bam 5-10/5-12 and Bam 3a + 3b) were shown to be stable for at least 4 years, the longest period between the isolations of the strains studied. When the stability of the 2 ("old" and "new") variants of the prototype (characterized by a slower and faster mobility of Bam fragment 5', respectively) was examined, we found that strains remained stable for at least 10 years (Fig.3). Therefore this marker seems to be suitable for further differentiation of strains when this is the only known difference.

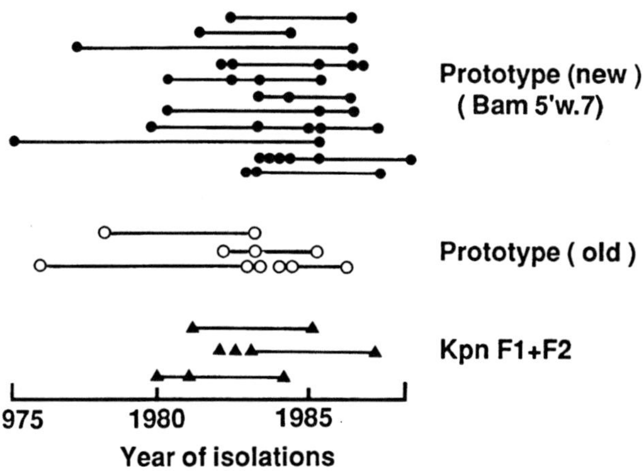

Fig. 3 Stability of DNA markers on farms. Symbols represent virus isolations (for explanations see text).

Based on the results of strains isolated with at least a 1-year-interval on 46 farms, we never did observe a change in the described markers of viruses from a particular farm, unless the whole pig population of the farm was replaced.

Geographical distribution of DNA markers

In Hungary the vast majority of ADV strains belongs to the prototype variant, namely the "new" version is found on 62% of the examined farms, while only 18% harbor the "old" variant of the prototype.

The "old prototype variant tends to cluster in some Eastern counties perhaps demonstrating the commercial activity of some large farms harboring this type of strains. This is even more apparent for viruses with the Kpn $F_1 + F_2$ marker. This is the dominant strain in a South-Eastern county: this variety was most likely distributed by a single farm in that region. This farm has been the major supplier for some years and now pigs on 11% of the farms in Hungary are infected with this strain.

The remaining 8 cleavage site markers were found on only 9% of the farms (a total of 27) examined. These varieties are randomly scattered in the country; perhaps they emerged later than those already widely spread in the country. Since reinfection of some AD-free herds was associated with strains with rare DNA markers the source of virus could be investigated.

Epidemiological investigations

We describe here, very briefly, some of the outbreaks where the origin of the virus and/or the mode of introduction of ADV strains were ascertained by RE analysis of their DNA.

1. AD appeared on a pig farm that had been negative for about 15 years. Movement of animals was excluded, but the farm had a feed mill. Grain and fodder were transported in and out of the plant in non-disinfected jute bags which had originated from other farms including some positive for AD. Several isolates from the farm were examined and all had a Kpn $F_1 + F_2$ marker. With the help of this DNA marker, unique in that region, we found among several possibilities the very farm from where this strain was introduced. Since the only relationship between the 2 places was restricted to feed transport, the actual mode of virus introduction was also proved (Nagy *et al.*, 1985a).

2. On 1 (A) of 2 farms that are located only some 500 meter apart, AD was eradicated by herd replacement and pigs were left unvaccinated. Within a year, clinical AD appeared on farm A and a rare DNA variety (Bam 3a + 3b) was isolated. On the adjacent farm (B), in spite of vaccination, sporadic AD cases (confirmed by virus isolation) could be observed from time to time. The strain colonizing farm B was also Bam 3a + 3b, thus confirming the source of virus of farm A, but not the mode of introduction, because no suspicious event could be singled out in this case (Nagy *et al.*, 1985b).

3. Farm L1 chose to eradicate by herd replacement after a series of AD outbreaks (from which Bam 5-10/5-12 varieties had been isolated). Breeding stock was purchased from a distant farm (Z) whose herd had been AD-free only for 2 years. A year after the repopulation of farm L1, AD broke out and strains were isolated with DNA marker Kpn $F_1 + F_2$ and with the prototype Bam pattern. So this strain was different from the one that had been isolated on the same farm before the eradication of AD. At this time, on the cooperative's other farm (L2), some kilometers away, where vaccination was still going on, also the Bam 5-10/5-12 variety was isolated. (This fact was in accordance with local evidence that formerly farm L1 had supplied pigs to farm L2). Therefore, farm L2 could not be the source of farm L1's new ADV strain. However, farm Z went also down with clinical AD, 1.5 year after the new outbreak on farm L1. DNA patterns (both by Bam and Kpn) of strains isolated on farm Z were identical with those of farm L1. Both farms were claimed to be epidemiologically closed, so one can speculate if virus was introduced to farm L1 by latently infected pigs purchased at farm Z (Nagy *et al.*, 1985c).

4. Farm N sold healthy vaccinated pigs to farm K located at the other part of the country. Clinical AD appeared in a few weeks on farm K and strains with unique marker (Kpn $C_1 + C_2$) were isolated. Farm N was singled out as the probable

supplier of this strain since this was the only other farm where the same marker had been found. Mode of virus introduction could be by latently infected pigs.

5. Vaccination crews carried out mass injection on farm X, populated with AD positive herd and located on one side of the river Danube. Within days they vaccinated on the other side of the river on farm Y, where AD broke out within 2 weeks after their visit. Here a strain with Bam 5-10/5-12 pattern was isolated. Anecdotal evidence pointed to farm X as a probable source of infection and indeed this notion was confirmed by checking the DNA pattern of a strain from our collection that had formerly been isolated on farm X.

The utility of DNA-fingerprinting was also evident in a number of cases when the origin of virus could not be determined, nevertheless epidemiological suspicions formed on the basis of e.g. anecdotal evidence could be excluded with the help of DNA-fingerprints of relevant virus strains.

DISCUSSION

RE analysis of the DNAs of ADV strains is a powerful tool to enable diagnosis to reveal genetic variations of virus strains. This information may complement diagnosis with data on the origin of the virus in particular outbreaks, and consequently its mode of the introduction as well. It is evident that epidemiological investigations should effectively contribute to the control of AD.

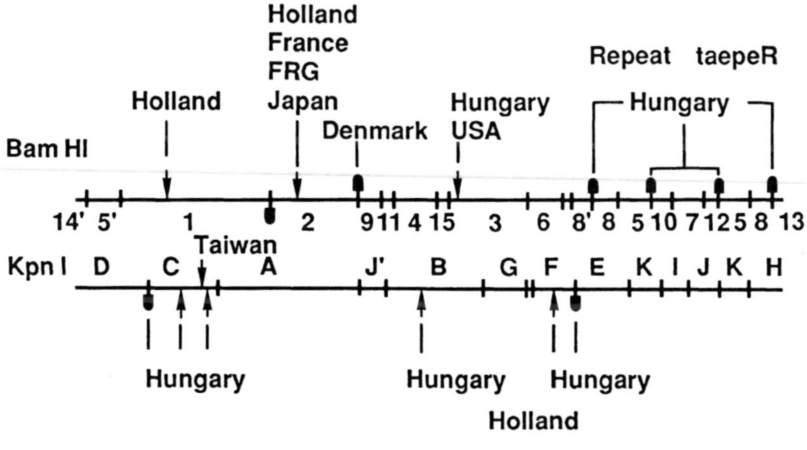

Fig. 4 Diversity of DNA cleavage site markers of ADV strains isolated worldwide (for references see text).

It became apparent during our studies that epidemiological investigations with any prospect of success can only be carried out if some requirements are met: a) there are suspicions based on local evidence (both anecdotal and written) as to the origin of the virus; b) epidemiological relationships of different locations can only be confirmed or excluded if representative virus strains are available from each place; c) there is large enough variability of genomes of strains belonging to epidemiologically unrelated outbreaks.

Variability of ADV strains has been studied by authors from various countries (for ref. see introduction). They examined some 400 to 500 strains isolated in different regions of the world (Western Europe, USA, Taiwan, Japan) and several markers based on cleavage site differences were described (Fig. 4). In Hungary we have found 9 rare cleavage site markers (Nagy *et al.*, 1985a, b, c), 7 of which were not reported elsewhere. One of these (Kpn $F_1 + F_2$) became dominant in a county most likely due to the commercial activity of a single breeder.

Long-term stability of some of the markers has been demonstrated in the field. Not only markers based on cleavage site differences proved to be stable for years on farms but a so-called variable one, involving the mobility of Bam fragment 5', proved also to be stable. Thus this marker, too, can be used for differentiation of strains.

We have taken advantage of the large number of strains that were available with supporting local data as to their origin, and epidemiological investigations were carried out in several cases of AD outbreaks. Conclusions pertaining to these studies are summarized below (Table 1).

TABLE 1 Utility of DNA-fingerprinting in epidemiological investigations in Hungary

1. Both ORIGIN of virus and MODE of introduction are ascertained
   - Indirect: a) Food bags
     - b) Iatrogenic:
       - movement of personnel from slaughterhouse
       - movement during mass vaccination
       - restraining procedure during blood-taking

   Direct : (Most likely) LATENTLY infected HEALTHY pigs purchased as
   - a) Unvaccinated ADV-free stock for repopulation
   - b) Vaccinated breeding stock

2. Only the ORIGIN of infection is ascertained
3. EXCLUSION of the suspicion of the origin of virus
4. Establishment of the FINGERPRINT of resident strains for post-eradication period

One has to add another possible benefit of knowing the DNA fingerprints of strains colonizing different farms. In the future when/if eradication will be carried out by selecting naturally infected animals from vaccinated herds, at failures one wants to know if AD reappeared due to the original (resident) strain of the farm or due to a newly introduced one.

REFERENCES

Ben-Porat, T., Deatly, A.M., Easterday, B.C., Galloway, D., Kaplan, A.S. and McGregor, S. 1984a. Latency of pseudorabies virus. Curr. Top. Vet. Med. Anim. Sci., **27**, 365-383. In: CEC Seminar on "Latent herpesvirus infections in veterinary medicine". (Eds. G. Wittmann, R.M. Gaskell and H.J. Rziha). (Martinus Nijhoff, The Hague).

Ben-Porat, T., Wu. C., Harper, L. and Lomniczi, B. 1984b. Biological significance of the alterations in restriction patterns of the genomes of different isolates of pseudorabies virus. In "Herpesvirus" (Ed. F. Rapp). UCLA Keystone Symposium. (A.R. Liss, Inc., New York). pp. 537-550.

Buchman, T.G., Simpson, T., Nosal, C. and Roizman, B. 1980. The structure of herpes simplex virus DNA and its application to molecular epidemiology. Ann. New York Acad. Sci., **354,** 279-290.

Clewley, J.P. and Bishop, D.H.L. 1982. Oligonucleotide fingerprinting of viral genomes. In "New Developments in Practical Virology" (Ed. C.R. Howard). (Alan R. Liss, Inc., New York). pp. 213-277.

Geck, P., Nagy, E. and Lomniczi, B. 1982. Differentiation of avirulent strains of Aujeszky's disease virus by restriction enzymes (in Hung.). Magy. Ao. Lapja, **37,** 651-656.

Gielkens, A.L.J. and Berns, A.J.M. 1982. Differentiation of Aujeszky's disease virus strains by restriction endonuclease analysis of the viral DNAs. Curr. Top. Vet. Med. Anim. Sci., **17,** 3-14. In: CEC Seminar on "Aujeszky's disease". (Eds. G. Wittmann and S.A. Hall). (Martinus Nijhoff, The Hague).

Gielkens, A.L.J., Van Oirschot, J.T., Van Schie, F.W. and Toma, B. 1984. Restriction endonuclease analysis of Aujeszky's disease virus DNA. In: CEC Seminar on "Recent Advances in Virus Diagnostics". (Eds. M.S McNulty and J.B. McFerran). (Martinus Nijhoff, The Hague). pp. 101-114.

Gielkens, A.L.J., van Oirschot, J.T. and Berns, A.J.M. 1985. Genome differences among field isolates and vaccine strains of pseudorabies virus. J. Gen. Virol., **66,** 69-82.

Hayward, G.S., Frenkel, N. and Roizman, B. 1975. Anatomy of herpes simplex virus DNA: Strain differences and heterogeneity in the locations of restriction endonuclease cleavage sites. Proc. Natl. Acad. Sci. USA, **72,** 1768-1772.

Herrmann, S.C., Heppner, B. and Ludwig, H. 1984. Pseudorabies viruses from clinical outbreaks and latent infections grouped into four major genome types. Curr. Top. Vet. Med. Anim. Sci., **27,** 387-402. In: CEC Seminar on "Latent herpesvirus infections in veterinary medicine". (Eds. G. Wittmann, R.M. Gaskell and H.J. Rziha). (Martinus Nijhoff, The Hague).

Lomniczi, B., Blankenship, M.L. and Ben-Porat, T. 1984. Deletions in the genomes of pseudorabies virus vaccine strains and existence of four isomers of the genomes. J. Virol., **49**, 970-979.

Ludwig, H., Heppner, B. and Herrmann, S. 1982. The genomes of different field isolates of Aujeszky's disease virus. Curr. Top. Vet. Anim. Sci., **17**, 15-22. In: CEC Seminar on "Aujeszky's disease". (Eds. G. Wittmann and S.A. Hall). (Martinus Nijhoff, The Hague).

Nagy, E. 1988. Differentiation of Aujeszky's disease virus strains by restriction enzyme analysis of their DNAs. Dissertation (Budapest).

Nagy, E., Máté, Zs., Kozaróczy, Gy., Szécsy, Sz. and Lomniczi, B. 1985a. Molecular epidemiology of Aujeszky's disease virus. I. Origin of the virus strain responsible for an outbreak on a disease-free farm in Borsod county (in Hung.). Magy. Ao. Lapja, **40**, 93-99.

Nagy, E., Palya, V., Vajda, G., Szécsy, Sz., Szigeti, S. and Lomniczi, B. 1985b. Molecular epidemiology of Aujeszky's disease virus. II. Characterization of virus strains and study of the epidemiological relationships in Csongrád county (in Hung.). Magy. Ao. Lapja, **40**, 597-601.

Nagy, E., Vajda, G., Végh, L., Szécsy, Sz. and Lomniczi, B. 1985c. Molecular epidemiology of Aujeszky's disease virus. III. Characterization of virus strains and study of the epidemiological relationships in Békés county (in Hung.). Magy. Ao. Lapja, **40**, 713-717.

Nishimori, T., Imada, T., Sakurai, M., Kitabayashi, T., Kawamura, H. and Nakajima, H. 1987. Restriction endonuclease analysis of Aujeszky's disease viruses isolated in Japan. Jap. J. Vet. Sci., **49**, 365-367.

Paul, P.S., Mengeling, W.L. and Pirtle, E.C. 1982. Differentiation of pseudorabies (Aujeszky's disease) virus strains by restriction endonuclease analysis. Arch. Virol., **73**, 193-198.

Pirtle, E.C., Wathen, M.W., Paul, P.S., Mengeling, W.L. and Sacks, J.M. 1984. Evaluation of field isolates of pseudorabies (Aujeszky's disease) virus as determined by restriction endonuclease analysis and hybridization. Am. J. Vet. Res., **45**,1906-1912.

Pritchett, R.F., Bush, C.E., Chang, T.J., Wang, J.T. and Zee, Y.C. 1984. Comparison of the genomes of pseudorabies (Aujeszky's disease) virus strains by restriction endonuclease analysis. Am. J. Vet. Res., **45**, 2486-2489.

Rixon, F.J. and Ben-Porat, T. 1979. Structural evolution of the DNA of pseudorabies-defective viral particles. Virol., **97**, 151-163.

Todd, D. and McFerran, J.B. 1985. Restriction endonuclease analysis of Aujeszky's disease (pseudorabies) virus DNA: Comparison of Northern Ireland isolates and isolates from other countries. Arch. Virol., **86**, 167-176.

SUMMARY

Two papers dealt with the development of vaccines against Aujeszky's disease. Eloit *et al.* presented first results on the construction of a recombinant adenovirus type 5 (Ad5) expressing the glycoprotein gp50 of pseudorabies virus (PRV). After infection of a human cell line permissive for Ad5, the expression of gp50 could be demonstrated on the cell surface by immunofluorescence. Experiments for the efficacy and in particular for pathogenic characteristics of the Ad5-PRV recombinant in swine are in progress.

The production, characterization and evaluation of PRV subunit vaccines was reported by Chappuis *et al.* The viral glycoproteins were prepared both from a wild-type virus and from a $gI^-/gp63^-$ deletion mutant. The glycoprotein content of the preparations was determined by measuring the amount of gII and gIII. The efficacy of both vaccines was equal. This subunit vaccine also conferred good protection to cats and dogs against wild-type PRV challenge infection. No correlation was observed between protection rate and titers of serum neutralizing antibodies of the vaccinated animals.

Rziha *et al.* reported first experiments concerning the latency characteristics of vaccine strains. The Begonia strain (gI^-/TK^-) appeared to replicate in neural tissues and tonsils to a markedly lesser extent than virulent PRV, and neither infectious virus was recoverable nor viral DNA could be detected after 4 months and immunosuppression. In swine vaccinated with strain NIA-4 (gI^-/TK^-) also no virus could be recovered 4 months after vaccination, although viral DNA was present in various tissues. NIA-4 vaccinated animals were not protected against a reactivable, latent infection after challenge with virulent PRV.

Jestin and Vannier presented different theoretical considerations on possible molecular events and biohazards which might happen after the application of genetically constructed products.

Finally, Lomniczi *et al.* presented results of a detailed DNA fingerprinting study of numerous PRV isolates circulating in Hungary during the last 13 years. Ten differentiable types of PRV could be classified by the use of distinct DNA marker fragments which proved to be stable in the field over many years. With the aid of those markers and additional supporting data on the circumstances of Aujeszky's disease outbreaks it was possible to trace the introduction and the "pathway" of the virus. Additionally, the data indicated that instability of some DNA fragments arising in cell culture cannot be easily extrapolated to instability *in vivo.*

J. T. van Oirschot (ed.), Vaccination and Control of Aujeszky's Disease, 103.

3. IMMUNE RESPONSES AGAINST PROTEINS OF AUJESZKY'S DISEASE VIRUS

Chairpersons J.T. van Oirschot and B. Toma

ROLE OF PSEUDORABIES VIRUS GLYCOPROTEINS IN IMMUNE RESPONSE

F.A. Zuckermann, T.C. Mettenleiter**, T. Ben-Porat**

*Department of Microbiology
Vanderbilt University School of Medicine
Nashville, Tennessee 37232
**Bundesforschungsanstalt für Viruskrankheiten der Tiere,
D 7400 Tübingen, FRG.

ABSTRACT

The role of the nonessential glycoproteins of pseudorabies virus (PRV) in immunity was assessed as follows: (1) The relative number of cytotoxic T lymphocytes (CTL) that were induced in mice inoculated with thymidine kinase minus (TK^-) virus that react with each of the glycoproteins was ascertained by using cells infected with virus mutants defective in one of these glycoproteins as target for lysis. (2) The role of the nonessential glycoproteins in eliciting neutralizing antibodies was determined. (3) The relative efficacy of the various PRV mutants defective in a given glycoprotein (as well as in TK activity, thereby rendering them avirulent) as vaccines was ascertained by assessing their ability to prevent mortality upon superinfection of immunized mice with virulent virus. The main conclusion drawn from the results obtained is as follows: Of the nonessential glycoproteins, gIII plays the most important role in immune response; mutants defective in the gIII gene were less effective in eliciting a cell-mediated response, as well as neutralizing antibodies. Furthermore, mutants defective in the TK gene, as well as in the gIII gene, did not confer as good a protection against challenge with virulent virus as did mutants defective in the TK gene and either the gI, gp63, of gX genes.

INTRODUCTION

Pseudorabies virus (PRV) is the etiological agent of Aujeszky's disease (AD), a disease that causes heavy economic losses to the swine industry. Eradication of the disease is of considerable economic importance throughout the world. Vaccination against AD with attenuated live vaccines isolated after passage in cell culture has been practiced for a number of years in many countries. More recently, genetically engineered avirulent strains have also been constructed as vaccines against PRV. In general, to reduce their virulence, the gene encoding the thymidine kinase (TK) has been deleted from these strains (Kit *et al.*, 1985; McGregor *et al.*, 1985). A defect in a nonessential viral glycoprotein is also sometimes introduced

J. T. van Oirschot (ed.), Vaccination and Control of Aujeszky's Disease, 107–117.

into these vaccine strains to facilitate the differentiation by serological means between animals that have been vaccinated only and animals that have been exposed to wild-type virus (Kit *et al.*, 1986; Van Oirschot *et al.*, 1986; Marchioli *et al.*, 1987).

It has been known for some time that vaccine strains defective in glycoproteins gI or gp63 (for example, the Bartha or Norden strains) can give rise to immunity and protect pigs from disease. It has also been shown that strains defective in either glycoprotein gIII or gX provide the animals with protection against challenge by wild-type virus (Kit *et al.*, 1986, Marchioli *et al.*, 1987). However, a comparison of the quality of the immunity produced by viruses which otherwise are isogenic but which are defective in one of these nonessential glycoproteins has not been assessed.

The aims of the studies presented in this paper were as follows: (1) to gain an understanding of the roles the various nonessential glycoproteins play in eliciting an immune response and (2) to compare the ability of otherwise isogenic PRV mutants which fail to express 1 of the nonessential viral glycoproteins to protect animals against challenge with virulent virus.

RESULTS

Role of PRV glycoproteins in cytotoxic T lymphocyte response

Mutants of PRV that are defective in the expression of 1 of the glycoproteins that are nonessential for virus replication in cell culture (gI$^-$, gIII$^-$, gp63$^-$ or gX$^-$) have been constructed in our laboratory. Fig. 1 illustrates the deletions that have been introduced into the genome of PRV(Ka) to inactivate the genes encoding the nonessential glycoproteins. The lack of synthesis of the appropriate glycoproteins in cells infected with the mutants was confirmed by immunoprecipitation followed by polyacrylamide gel electrophoresis (PAGE) (data not shown). These mutants provide an opportunity to assess the relative intensity of the cell-mediated and humoral immune responses that each of these glycoproteins induces under natural conditions, i.e., in animals infected with live PRV. These virions can also be used to compare the efficacy as vaccines of mutants that are defective in 1 of these glycoproteins but are otherwise isogenic.

The role of each nonessential glycoprotein of PRV in cell-mediated immunity can be ascertained by comparing the ability of CTLs to lyse cells infected with either wild-type virus or with a mutant defective in the expression of 1 of these glycoproteins. However, it was first necessary to determine whether these glycoproteins are expressed on the surface of the cells. This was done by flow cytofluorometry and antibody-dependent complement mediated cell lysis. The results obtained (data not shown) showed that gI and gIII (nonessential glycoproteins) are expressed on the cell surface as abundantly as is gII (an essential glycoprotein).

However, the cell surface did not react with the monoclonal antibodies against gp63 that we had at our disposal (a generous gift from Dr. P. Desmettre, Rhône Mérieux) nor did we have appropriate antibodies against gX (data not shown). Thus, although it is clear that gI and gIII are expressed on the cell surface, we do not know whether gp63 and gX are.

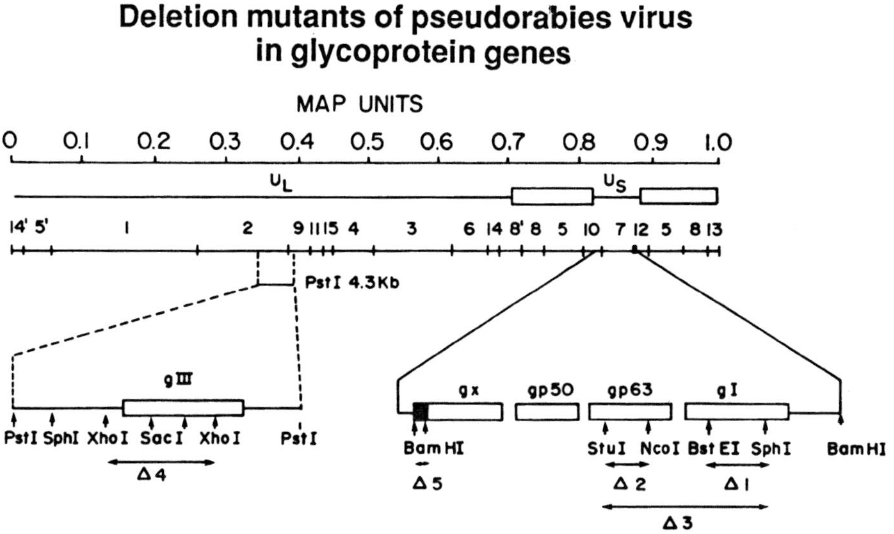

Fig. 1 The top of the figure indicates the Bam HI restriction map of PRV DNA. The positions of the genes are indicated on line 4. The sequences in the genes that span the deletions are indicated by horizontal arrows. Δ1, Δ2, Δ3, and Δ4 are deletion mutants. Δ5 is a deletion/insertion mutant into which the Hae III fragment of M13 containing the multiple cloning site has been introduced.

CTL response to PRV was induced in DBA/2 mice by injection of a TK^- mutant of PRV(Ka) in the foot pads. Lymphocytes were isolated from the draining popliteal lymph nodes 6 days after immunization and were cultured for 3 days. These lymphocytes were able to lyse PRV-infected, but not uninfected, and syngeneic, but not allogenic cells, indicating that they are major histocompatibility complex restricted. Furthermore, the anti-PRV activity was associated with cells that were Thy 1^+, Lyt 2^+, $L3T4^-$, indicating that they were CTLs (data not shown).

To determine the relative role that each nonessential PRV glycoprotein plays in the reactivity of anti-PRV CTLs with PRV-infected cells, the ability of the former to lyse syngeneic cells infected with wild-type virus or with mutants into which deletions in the genes encoding gI and gp63, gX of gIII have been introduced (see Fig. 1), was compared. The specific lysis of target cells infected with the double mutant gI⁻/gp63⁻ or with the gX⁻ mutant was the same as that of cells infected with wild-type virus (Fig. 2), suggesting that CTLs against glycoproteins gI, gp63, and gX do not contribute significantly to the overall reactivity of the anti-PRV CTLs. In contrast, the effector: target ratio needed to obtain comparable specific lysis with gIII⁻-infected cells was significantly higher than that for wild-type infected cells. Effector: target ratios required to lyse 30% of the cells varied somewhat in different experiments. In 4 different experiments it was 50:1, 32:1, 21:1 and 15:1 for gIII- mutant infected cells and 10:1, 5:1, 12:1 and 7:1 for wild-type infected cells. These results suggest that a significant proportion of the anti-PRV CTL reactivity was directed against gIII.

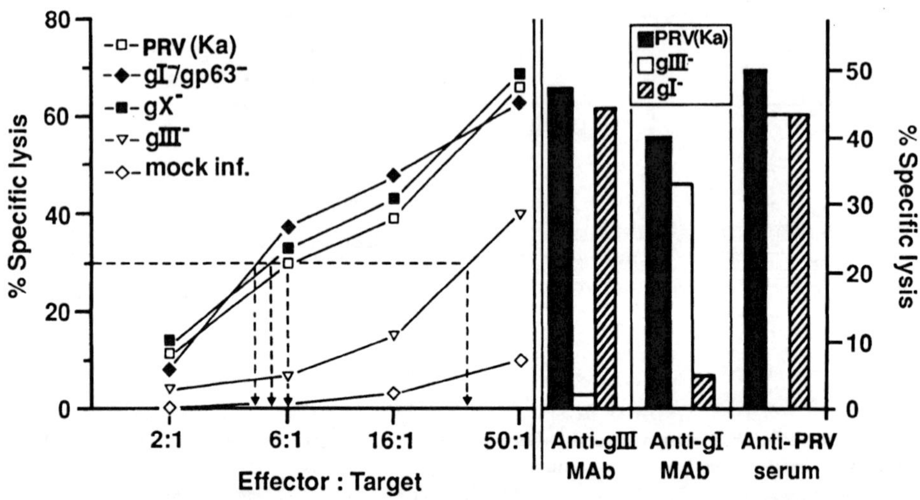

Fig. 2 Role of PRV nonessential glycoproteins in eliciting cytotoxic T lymphocytes. Left panel: Mouse embryo cells transformed by SV40 (MESV) (H-2d) were infected (MOI = 10 PFU/cell) with wild-type PRV or with PRV glycoprotein deletion mutants defective in the expression of gI and gp63 (gI⁻/gp63⁻), gX (gX⁻) or gIII (gIII⁻). At 10 h post infection, part of the cells were used in a ^{51}Cr-release assay (4 h) with anti-PRV CTLs generated in DBA/2 mice. Right Panel: Part of the same infected cells were also incubated for 1 h either with anti-PRV serum or with monoclonal antibodies against gI or gIII, followed by an additional hour of incubation with rabbit complement. The percent specific lysis was determined.

To rule out the possibility that the lower CTL activity obtained against gIII⁻-infected cells was due to a lower susceptibility to lysis of these cells, their sensitivity to anti-PRV antibodies and complement was also tested. Lysis of wild-type PRV(Ka), gI⁻/gp63⁻ or gIII⁻-infected cells was similar (Fig. 2). As expected, anti-gIII monoclonal antibody (MAb) did not lyse the cells infected with gIII⁻ virus, whereas anti-gI MAb did. Similarly, anti-gI MAb did not lyse cells infected with a gI⁻ mutant, but anti-gIII MAb did.

That a large proportion of the CTLs induced against PRV are directed against gIII was also established by assessing the ability of cells infected with these mutants to stimulate an *in vitro* secondary CTL response. The rationale for this experiment was that CTLs specific against gIII would not be antigen-stimulated by stimulator cells that lack gIII and a smaller number of lytic units should be observed in gIII⁻ stimulated than wild-type stimulated CTL cultures. The difference in the number of lytic units obtained after stimulation with cells infected with wild-type virus or with a gIII⁻ mutant should provide an estimate of the importance of gIII in CTL response. Furthermore, in this experiment, the same target cells were used and possible differences in the susceptibility of the target cells to lysis were therefore eliminated as a source of variability.

Cells obtained from the popliteal and sacral lymph node of mice which had been immunized in the foot pad 4 weeks previously with TK⁻ PRV were restimulated in vitro with splenic adherent cells infected with either wild-type PRV(Ka) or with mutants defective in the synthesis of a glycoprotein and tested against wild-type infected target cells. Mock-infected splenic adherent cells served as controls for background anti-PRV CTL activity. The results (Fig. 3) showed that the relative number of CTLs able to lyse PRV-infected cells was the same when the population of CTLs obtained from PRV-immunized mice was restimulated with wild-type PRV and a gI⁻/gp63⁻ mutant. Similar results were also obtained with a gX⁻ mutant (data not shown). However, the number of CTLs able to lyse PRV-infected cells was considerably lower when the CTL population had been restimulated with a gIII⁻ mutant of PRV.

The experiments summarized in Figs. 2 and 3 indicate that a relatively large proportion of the anti-PRV CTLs is directed against gIII. Glycoprotein gIII is a homolog of glycoprotein gC of HSV (Robbins *et al.*, 1986). It has been reported that glycoprotein gC of HSV is the immunodominant antigen eliciting CTLs in mice (Glorioso *et al.*, 1985; Kümel *et al.*, 1985; Rosenthal *et al.*, 1987). Thus, the homologous proteins of HSV and PRV behave similarly in this respect.

Role of nonessential PRV glycoproteins in eliciting neutralizing antibodies

We have reported previously that while a relatively large part of the neutralizing antibodies present in pooled convalescent sera obtained from pigs are directed against gIII, antibodies against gI play little or no role in neutralization (Ben-Porat *et al.*, 1986). The lack of neutralizing antibodies against gI/gp63 and the presence of neutralizing antibodies against gIII in pooled convalescent serum of swine were confirmed by the results summarized in Table 1. Bartha is not as susceptible to the antiserum as is PRV(Ka). After restoration to Bartha of the gI and gp63 gene derived from PRV(Ka) (Bartha 43/25a), no significant increase in susceptibility to the anti-serum was observed. However, after replacement of the Bartha gIII gene ($gIII^{B}$), which is atypical and behaves in an abnormal manner (Ben-Porat *et al.*, 1986; Mettenleiter *et al.*, 1988), with a gIII gene derived from PRV(Ka) ($gIII^{Ka}$), the variant Bartha (Bartha 43/25a-$gIII^{+}$) became almost as susceptible to neutralization by the pooled convalescent serum as PRV(Ka).

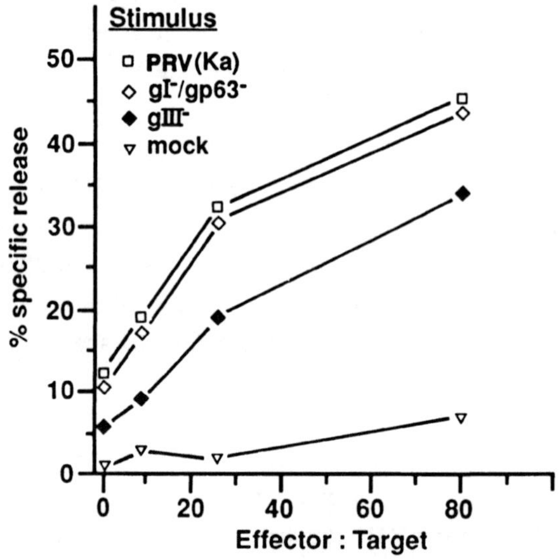

Fig. 3 Ability of cells infected with deletion mutants defective in nonessential glycoproteins to induce a secondary anti-PRV cytotoxic T lymphocyte response. Lymph node cells were isolated from DBA/2 mice 4 weeks after immunization in the foot pad with PRV TK⁻. They were cocultured for 5 days with irradiated (2500 R) syngeneic splenic adherent cells that had been either mock-infected, infected with wild-type PRV, with a deletion mutant defective in the expression of gI and gp63 ($gI^-/gp63^-$), or a deletion mutant defective in the expression of gIII ($gIII^-$). Their ability to lyse PRV-infected syngeneic cells was then ascertained in a ^{51}Cr-release assay.

Immunity of animals vaccinated with TK⁻ mutants defective in gI, gp63, gIII or gX

Because animals infected with PRV will probably respond to many viral proteins with humoral, as well as cell-mediated, immunity, it is probable that most vaccines, including those that lack 1 or more glycoproteins, will provide some protection. The degree of protection provided by different deletion mutants may vary, however. Not only is the direct role of each glycoprotein in eliciting immunity important, but also the deletion of a glycoprotein may affect the ability of a vaccine strain to replicate *in vivo* which in turn will determine the intensity of the immune response.

TABLE 1 Neutralization of Bartha variants with convalescent pig serum

Virus variant	Phenotype	Pig convalescent serum (% survival)
PRV(Ka)	$gI^{+}/gp63^{+}/gIII^{Ka}$	3[a]
Bartha	$gI^{-}/gp63^{-}/gIII^{B}$	78
Bartha $gIII^{Ka}$	$gI^{-}/gp63^{-}/gIII^{Ka}$	8
Bartha 43/25a	$gI^{+}/gp63^{+}/gIII^{B}$	72
Bartha 43/25a-$gIII^{Ka}$	$gI^{+}/gp63^{+}/gIII^{Ka}$	6

[a]Approximately 200 PFU of each virus mutant was incubated for 60 min at 37°C with heat-inactivated pooled pig anti-PRV convalescent serum (final concentration, 1:500; a generous gift from Dr. D.

We have ascertained the potency as vaccines of PRV mutants that differ only in that they are defective in different nonessential glycoproteins (i.e., which are otherwise isogenic) against various doses of challenge with wild-type virus. The aim of these experiments was to assess the importance of each of the nonessential glycoproteins in eliciting immunity under conditions which mimic those of natural infection, i.e., infection with live virus strains.

Each of the mutants defective in a nonessential glycoprotein was rendered avirulent by inactivation of the TK gene, as described previously (McGregor *et al.*, 1985). Groups of ICR mice (30 each) were vaccinated with either the parental PRV(Ka)TK^{-} virus or with TK^{-} mutants that were also defective in either gX, gI or gIII. Four weeks after vaccination the animals were challenged with different doses of wild-type virulent PRV(Ka) and the number of vaccinated animals, as well as unvaccinated controls, that died, was determined (Fig. 4).

The difference in the protection afforded to mice by vaccination with wild-type (TK^{-}) virions or TK^{-} mutants that failed to express either gI or gX was relatively small. It was interesting to note that gI^{-} mutants appeared almost as protective as wild-type virus despite the fact that gI^{-} mutants do not replicate as well locally in mice as does wild-type virus (L. Zsak, F.A. Zuckermann and T. Ben-Porat, manuscript in preparation). The most salient observation, however, to emerge from these experiments was that the $gIII^{-}$ mutant appeared to be significantly less effective in providing protection against challenge with wild-type virus than were the other mutants.

The immunized mice were also bled prior to challenge and the neutralizing activity of their sera against PRV was ascertained. All sera possessed neutralizing activity but the sera of mice immunized with the TK⁻ gIII⁻ virions had between 10-100 fold lower neutralizing titers than did mice immunized either with wild-type (TK⁻) virus or with the TK⁻ mutants that were also defective in gX or gI/gp63 (data not shown).

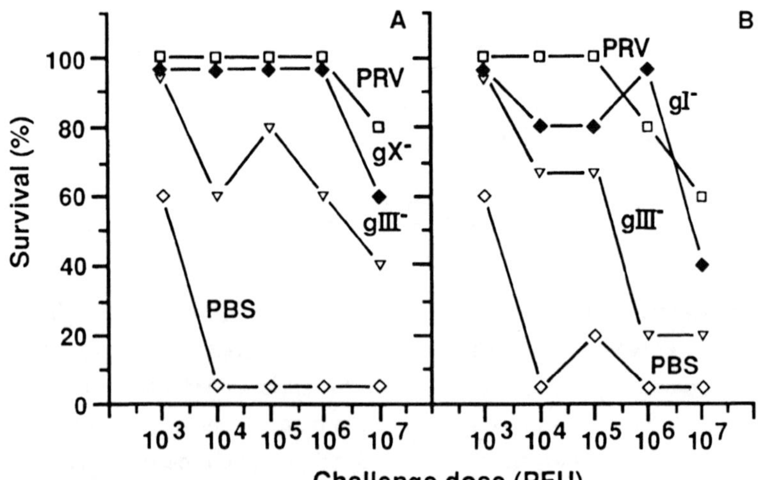

Fig. 4 Protection of mice against challenge with wild-type virus by vaccination with gI⁻, gX⁻ or gIII⁻ mutants. ICR mice were immunized intramuscularly with 6×10^3 (A), or 6×10^4 (B) PFU of TK⁻ strains of PRV defective in the indicated glycoproteins. Four weeks later the animals were challenged intraperitoneally with the indicated doses of wild-type PRV and the percent of surviving mice was recorded. PRV = PRV(Ka)TK⁻; gX⁻ = PRV(Ka)TK⁻gX⁻; gIII⁻ = PRV(Ka)TK⁻gIII⁻; gI⁻ = PRV(Ka)TK⁻gI⁻; PBS = phosphate buffered saline (dilution medium).

DISCUSSION

We have ascertained the relative importance of 4 different nonessential glycoproteins in immune response. Our results show that PRV gIII, but not gI, gp63 and gX, plays a significant role in eliciting CTLs. A major part of the neutralizing antibody present in convalescent pig serum is also directed against gIII. Furthermore, mutants that do not express gIII are significantly less effective in protecting mice against challenge with virulent virus than are mutants that do not express either gX, gI or gp63. The latter appear to be almost as effective in protection tests as is virus that expressed these glycoproteins. That gX does not confer protection against challenge with PRV has been previously reported (Thomsen *et al.*, 1987).

Control of PRV infections in swine can, in principle, be achieved by approaches that couple eradication of the infectious agent with vaccination. However, for the program of eradication and vaccination to be compatible, it is essential to be able to distinguish between animals that have been vaccinated and those that have been exposed to a field strain of the virus. To this end, strains which do not express 1 (or several) nonessential viral proteins have been and are being constructed to provide a means of distinguishing serologically the vaccinated animals from animals exposed to field strains. Since latent infections are important in perpetuating the disease, it is essential that a vaccine be sufficiently potent not only to protect against disease but also to prevent the establishment of latency in vaccinated animals that have come in contact with superinfecting virulent strains. It is likely that the more immunogenic a vaccine, the better it will be able to prevent the establishment of such latent infections. It is important, therefore, that the most immunogenic vaccines be identified.

We show here that gIII plays an important role in the immune response of animals and in their protection against challenge with wild-type virus. On the other hand, we found that gI, gp63 or gX are much less important. The relatively poor protection that the gIII$^-$ virus affords the animals, as well as the low level of neutralizing antibodies it induces in the vaccinated animals, can be ascribed, at least in part, to the importance of gIII as an immunogen. However, it could also be due to the reduced ability of the gIII$^-$ virus to replicate in the animal. Glycoprotein gIII has been shown to be multifunctional; it plays a pivotal role in virus adsorption (Schreurs *et al.*, 1988) and also affects virus release (Mettenleiter *et al.*, 1988; Whealy *et al.*, 1988). The less efficient replication of the gIII$^-$ mutants could contribute to the lower level of protection it affords the animals.

Whatever the basis for the relatively poor protection the gIII$^-$ mutant affords the animals, it is clear that the deletion of this glycoprotein from vaccine strains may not be advisable.

ACKNOWLEDGEMENTS

This investigation was supported by a grant (AI-10947) from the National Institutes of Health. Thomas C. Mettenleiter was supported by a fellowship (Me 854/1-2(4) from the Deutsche Forschungsgemeinschaft. Federico A. Zuckermann was supported by Public Health Service training grant 5T32-CA09385 from the National Cancer Institute.

REFERENCES

Ben-Porat, T., DeMarchi, J.M., Lomniczi, B. and Kaplan, A.S. 1986. Role of glycoproteins of pseudorabies virus in eliciting neutralizing antibodies. Virol., **154,** 325-334.

Glorioso, J., Kees, U., Kümel, G., Kirchner, H. and Krammer, P.H. 1985. Identification of herpes simplex virus type 1 (HSV-1) glycoprotein gC as the immunodominant antigen for HSV-1-specific memory cytotoxic T lymphocytes. J. Immunol., **135,** 575-582.

Kit, S., Kit, M. and Pirtle, E.C. 1985. Attenuated properties of thymidine kinase-negative deletion mutants of PRV. Am. J. Vet. Res., **46,** 1359-1367.

Kit, S., Sheppard, M., Ichimura, H. and Kit, M. 1986. Second-generation pseudorabies virus vaccine with deletions in thymidine kinase and glycoprotein genes. Am. J. Vet. Res., **48,** 780-793.

Kümel, G., Kaerner, H.C., Levine, M., Schröder, C.H. and Glorioso, J. 1985. Passive immune protection by herpes simplex virus-specific monoclonal antibodies and monoclonal antibody-resistant mutants altered in pathogenicity. J. Virol., **56,** 930-937.

Marchioli, C.C., Yancey, R.J., Wardley, R.C. Thomson, D.R. and Post, L.E. 1987. A vaccine strain of pseudorabies virus with deletions in the thymidine kinase and glycoprotein X genes. Am. J. Vet. Res., **48,** 1577-1583.

McGregor, S., Easterday, B.C., Kaplan, A.S. and Ben-Porat, T. 1985. Vaccination of swine with thymidine kinase deficient mutants of pseudorabies virus. Am. J. Vet. Res., **46,** 1494-1497.

Mettenleiter, T.C., Schreurs, C., Zuckermann, F.A., Ben-Porat, T. and Kaplan, A.S. 1988. Role of glycoprotein gIII of pseudorabies virus in virulence. J. Virol., **62,** 2712-1717.

Robbins, A.K., Watson, R.J., Whealy, M.E., Hays, W.W. and Enquist, L.W. 1986. Characterization of a pseudorabies virus glycoprotein gene with homology to herpes simplex virus type 1 and type 2 glycoprotein C. J. Virol., **58,** 339-347.

Rosenthal, K.L., Smiley, J.R., South, S. and Johnson, D.C. 1987. Cells expressing herpes simplex virus glycoprotein gC but not gB, gD or gE are recognized by murine virus-specific cytotoxic T lymphocytes. J. Virol., **61,** 2438-2447.

Schreurs, C., Mettenleiter, T.C., Zuckermann, F.A., Sugg, N. and Ben-Porat, T. 1988. Glycoprotein gIII of pseudorabies virus is multifunctional. J. Virol., **62,** 2251-2257.

Thomsen, D.R., Marchioli, C.C., Yancey, R.J. and Post, L.E. 1987. Replication and virulence of pseudorabies virus mutants lacking glycoprotein gX. J. Virol., **61,** 229-232.

Van Oirschot, J.T., Rziha, H.J., Moonen, P.J.L.M., Pol, J.M.A. and Van Zaane, D. 1986. Differentiation of serum antibodies from pigs vaccinated or infected with Aujeszky's disease virus by a competitive immunoassay. J. Gen. Virol., **67,** 1179-1182.

Whealy, M.E., Robbins, A.K. and Enquist, L.W. 1988. Pseudorabies virus glycoprotein gIII is required for efficient growth in tissue culture. J. Virol., **62,** 2512-2515.

DIFFERENTIATION BETWEEN PIGS INFECTED BY AUJESZKY'S DISEASE VIRUS AND PIGS VACCINATED WITH gI-NEGATIVE STRAINS

M. Eloit, D. Fargeaud**, P. Vannier***, B. Toma**

*Institut National de la Recherche Agronomique
Laboratoire d'Epidémiologie et de Physiopathologie des maladies à virus
7 avenue du Général de Gaulle, 94704 Maisons-Alfort cedex, France
**Rhône Mérieux, 245 rue Marcel Mérieux, 69007 Lyon, France
***Station de Pathologie Porcine, Les Croix, 22440 Ploufragan, France

ABSTRACT

A competitive ELISA which allows the detection of antibodies against glycoprotein I (gI) and glycoprotein III of Aujeszky's disease virus was tested with sera collected in the field. No false positive result arose when sera from fattening pigs free of Aujeszky's disease, vaccinated or not with gI-negative strains, were examined. A study conducted in pigs infected and/or vaccinated with gI-positive strains led to the conclusion that the competitive ELISA was at least as sensitive as a commercially available indirect ELISA. An epidemiological survey conducted in Brittany in 45 fattening herds vaccinated with a gI-negative strain allowed to detect at least 6 infected herds.

INTRODUCTION

Since 2 years, information about the structure of Aujeszky's disease virus (ADV) has shown that some vaccinal strains (i.e. Bartha, NIA-4, Norden) do not express glycoprotein (gI) (Mettenleiter *et al.*, 1985; Ben-Porat *et al.*, 1986). This feature led our team, like others (Van Oirschot *et al.*, 1986; Van Oirschot and De Waal, 1987) to develop a competitive immunoassay which allows one to detect gI antibodies in swine sera.

First good results were obtained on experimentally vaccinated and/or infected pigs (Eloit *et al.*, 1988a,b). We report here on the use of this test under field conditions in different fattening herds: a herd neither vaccinated nor infected; an Aujeszky's disease (AD) free herd vaccinated with a gI-negative (gI^-) strain; herds vaccinated with a gI-positive (gI^+) strain located in an area (Brittany) with high AD prevalence; herds vaccinated with a gI^- strain in the same area.

J. T. van Oirschot (ed.), Vaccination and Control of Aujeszky's Disease, 119–127.

MATERIALS AND METHODS

ELISA tests

The competitive enzyme immunoassay has been described (Eloit *et al.*, 1988a). Briefly, each serum to be tested was incubated with solubilized glycoproteins from potassium tartrate gradient purified virions. After 3 washes, an anti gI monoclonal antibody was added, then bound antibodies were probed with a biotin labelled antimouse IgG (H + L) serum. The reaction was developed with streptavidin-peroxidase and OPD as substrate. To give a reference, each serum was also tested, in the same manner, against an anti glycoprotein III (gIII) monoclonal antibody.

For each serum, the inhibition ratio (I) was calculated as follows:

$$I = \left(1 - \frac{\text{OD serum}}{\text{OD negative standard}}\right) \times 100$$

The gI antibody responses were scored as positive when they were greater than 40%, and scored as doubtful when they ranged between 30 and 40%. The gIII antibody responses were scored as positive when they were greater than 30%.

In some cases, a commercially available indirect ELISA, widely used in diagnostic laboratories in France, was used (Enzygnost Aujeszky, Behringwerke).

Sera

Exp 1: Forty-nine sera were collected in a fattening herd, free of ADV. The pigs were not vaccinated.

Exp 2: Fifty-eight fattening pigs (110 days old), located in an area free of AD, were vaccinated with the Bartha strain (Suvaxyn Aujeszky, Salsbury). Blood samples were taken at the slaughterhouse 1.5 months later.

Exp 3: Forty-six fattening pigs or sows were sampled at the slaughterhouse of Lamballe (Brittany). In this area, which is highly infected by ADV, vaccination of herds with gI^+ strains was widely used, so we hoped to collect most sera containing antibodies to gI.

Exp 4: Fifteen 3-month-old fattening pigs, born of sows vaccinated with a gI^+ strain (Geskypur, Rhône Mérieux), were vaccinated with a gI^- strain (Auskimune K, Norden). Two months later, at the end of the fattening period, the pigs were bled.

Exp 5: In a recent epidemiological survey in Brittany, 45 fattening herds vaccinated with a gI^- strain (Suvaxyn Aujeszky, Salsbury) were studied. The pigs have been vaccinated when they were 2.5 to 3-month-old. Blood samples were taken from 10 pigs in each herd. At the time of sampling, pigs were 130 to 150-day-old.

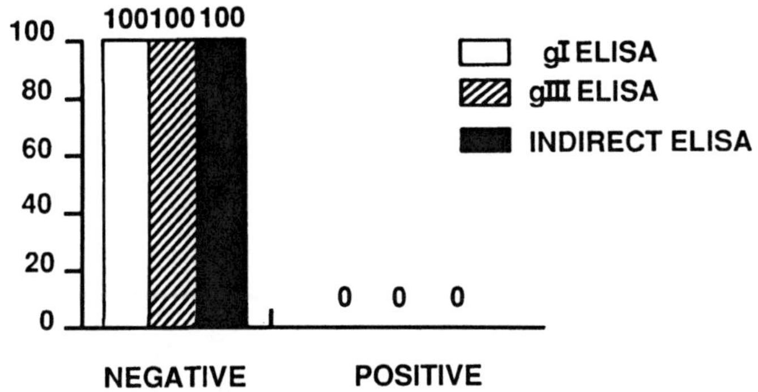

Fig. 1 Experiment 1: 49 pigs were sampled in a nonvaccinated fattening herd, free of Aujeszky's disease. Blood samples were tested by the competitive ELISAs and a commercial indirect ELISA. Percentages of positive (or doubtful) and negative results are shown.

RESULTS

Specificity

The results of experiments 1 and 2 are summarized in Fig. 1 and 2, respectively. No antibodies against gI or gIII could be detected in pigs which were neither infected nor vaccinated (Fig. 1). Only antibodies against gIII developed in pigs vaccinated with the Bartha strain (Fig. 2).

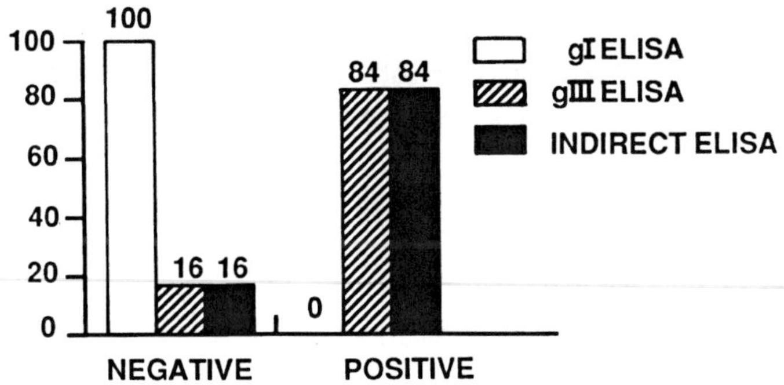

Fig 2. Experiment 2: 58 fattening pigs (110-day-old) were vaccinated with the Bartha strain. Blood samples were taken 1.5 months later and tested by the competitive ELISAs and a commercial indirect ELISA. Percentages of positive (or doubtful) and negative results are shown.

Detectability

Our competitive ELISA was compared to a commercially available indirect ELISA widely used in France. The gIII competitive ELISA is quite as sensitive as the indirect

ELISA, as shown by the results from experiments 2 and 3 (Fig. 2 and 3, respectively). Results of gI ELISA are summarized in Fig. 3: the ratio of positive or doubtful pigs was 74%, whereas indirect ELISA gave a 63% ratio. We assume that this difference originates from a better detectability of our competitive ELISA, and is not a consequence of a lack of specificity, as shown in experiments 1 and 2.

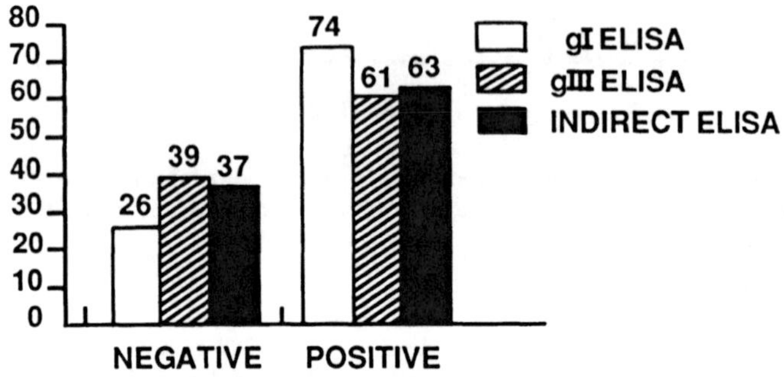

Fig. 3 Experiment 3: 46 fattening pigs and sows were sampled at the slaughterhouse of Lamballe. Most of them were presumably vaccinated with gI^{+} strains. Blood samples were tested by the competitive ELISAs and a commercial indirect ELISA. Percentages of positive (or doubtful) and negative results are shown.

Epidemiological survey

An epidemiological survey of AD in Brittany has been going on for the first months of 1988. As a part of this study, we tested with our competitive ELISA 45 fattening herds which had been previously vaccinated with gI^{-} strains.

Since in this area sows were vaccinated with gI^{+} strains, it was necessary to conduct a preliminary experiment to investigate potential interference of residual colostral antibodies against gI: several litters of pigs born of sows vaccinated with a gI^{+} strain were tested at the beginning and at the end of the fattening period. Fig. 4 (experiment 4) shows typical results from this kind of experiment: gIII antibody responses after vaccination were better in pigs with low levels of colostral antibodies at the time of vaccination; colostral gI antibodies can persist in 5-month-old pigs, especially in those which showed high levels of gI antibodies when they were 3-month-old. This persistence led to doubtful responses (between 30 and 40%) in 8 pigs. Thus, for the epidemiological study, only gI responses above 40% were taken into account.

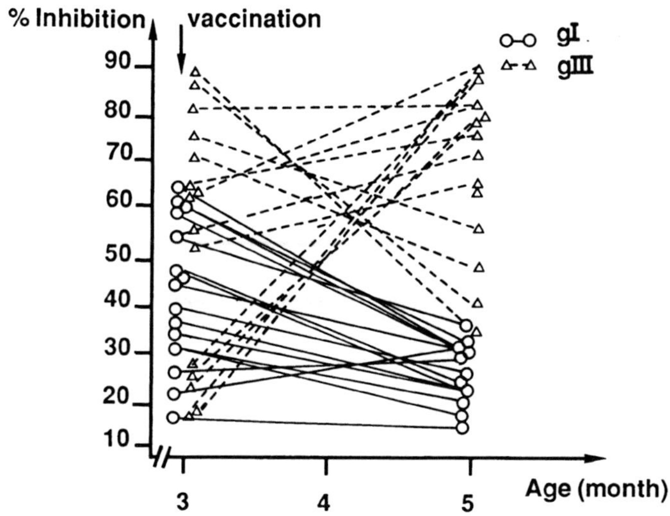

Fig. 4 Experiment 4: 15 3-month-old fattening pigs, born of sows vaccinated with a gI^{+} strain, were vaccinated with a gI^{-} strain. Blood samples were taken 2 months later and tested with the competitive ELISAs.

The results of the epidemiological survey are summarized in Table 1. Herds were quoted doubtful in all the cases where we got positive results without knowledge of the age of the pigs, because interference of colostral antibodies could not be eliminated.

TABLE 1 Epidemiological survey: summary of the results

Infected	Doubtful	Free
6	4	35

Fig. 5 to 8 show typical results from some herds. No infected pigs could be detected in herd 17900 (Fig. 5). Most infected herds which were detected looked like herd 17828 (Fig. 6), where a large part of the pigs were infected. In herd 17876 (Fig. 7) only a few animals were infected. In the case of herd 17809 (Fig. 8) 1 pen was infected (left part of the picture), whereas the other was probably free of ADV (right part of the picture).

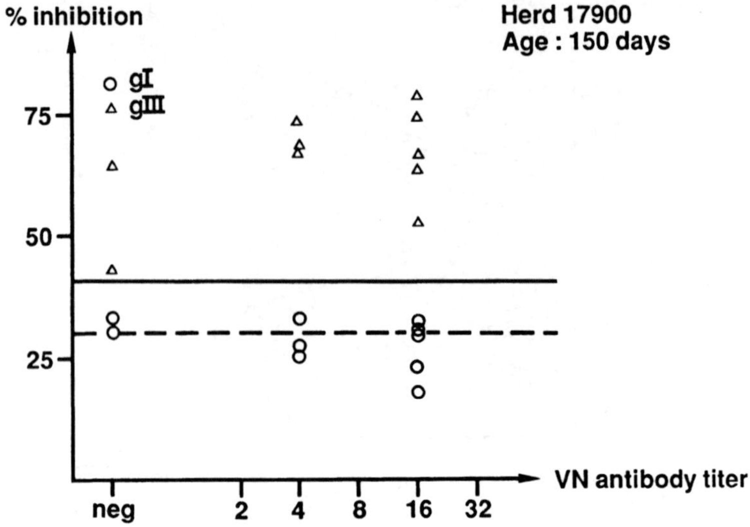

Fig. 5 Epidemiological survey (herd 17900): correspondence between virus-neutralizing antibody titers and antibody responses to gI and gIII.

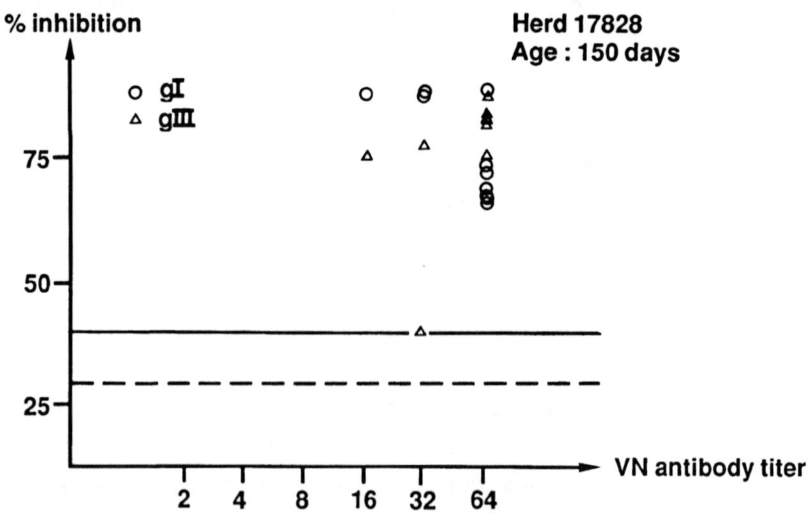

Fig. 6 Epidemiological survey (herd 17828): correspondence between virus-neutralizing antibody titers and antibody responses to gI and gIII.

DISCUSSION

We have recently described a competitive ELISA which allows the titration of antibodies against gI and gIII of ADV in pig sera (Eloit *et al.*, 1988a,b). This report extends those first findings by demonstrating that this test is suitable under field conditions. In experiments 1 and 2, no false positive result arises from pigs free of AD, vaccinated or not with gI$^-$ strains. Experiment 3 shows that the gI- ELISA was at least as sensitive as a commercially available indirect ELISA widely used in France. Besides, unpublished results indicate that the gI- and gIII-ELISA were sensitive enough to detect the EC reference serum diluted 1/4 to 1/8.

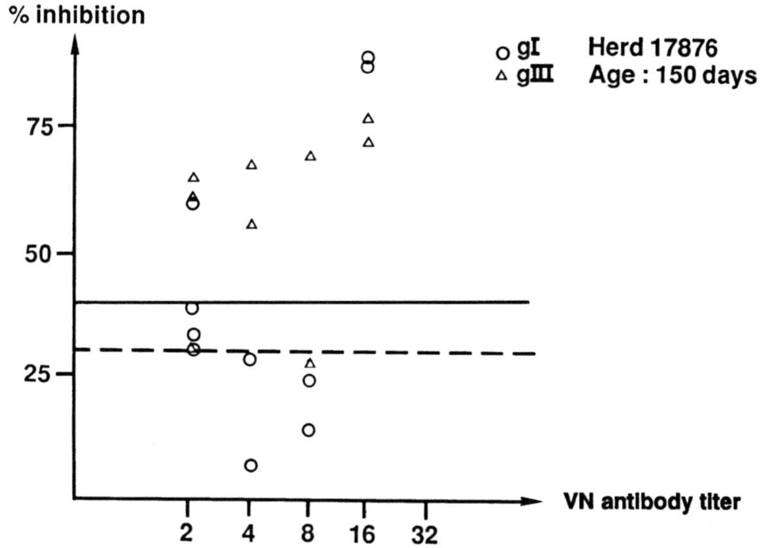

Fig. 7 Epidemiological survey (herd 17876): correspondence between virus-neutralizing antibody titers and antibody responses to gI and gIII.

We used the gI and gIII competitive ELISA in an epidemiological survey conducted in fattening herds in Brittany. These pigs were born to sows vaccinated with gI$^+$ strains and exhibited residual amounts of colostral antibodies against gI, even at the end of the fattening period (experiment 4). Nevertheless, we were able to detect at least 6 (and perhaps 10) infected herds, with variable pig infection rates in each herd.

These results show that this kind of test can be used in epidemiological surveys in areas where herds are vaccinated with gI$^-$ strains: the knowledge of herd infection rates will permit to choose the right moment to stop vaccination of herds. Besides, in breeding herds, the competitive ELISA would permit to selectively slaughter infected sows. The problem is quite different in fattening herds where knowledge of infected herds is only of epidemiological interest.

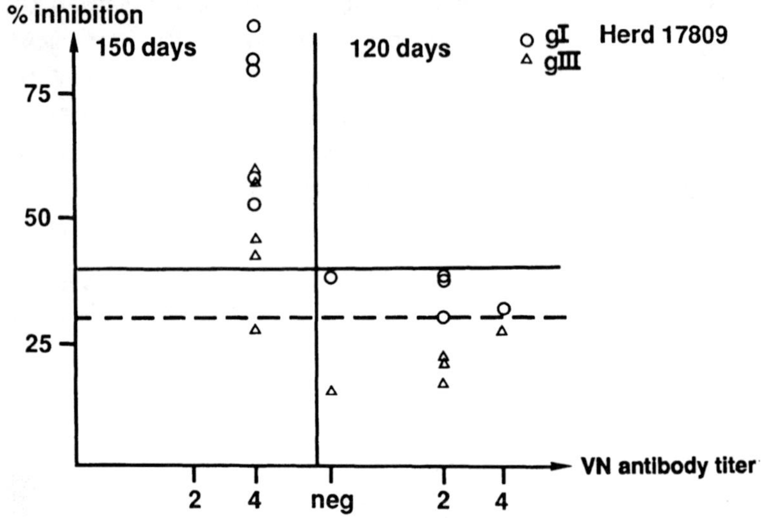

Fig. 8 Epidemiological survey (herd 17809): correspondence between virus-neutralizing antibody titers and antibody responses to gI and gIII. Two groups of pigs (respectively on the left and right part of the picture) are shown.

ACKNOWLEDGEMENTS

We thank Mrs. M. Andriamanga and Mrs. A. Fournier for their excellent technical assistance.

REFERENCES

Ben-Porat, T., Demarchi, J., Pendrys, J., Veach, R.A. and Kaplan, A.S. 1986. Proteins specified by the short unique region of the genome of pseudorabies virus play a role in the release of virions from certain cells. J. Virol., **57,** 191-196.

Eloit, M., Fargeaud, D., Vannier, P. and Toma, B. 1988a. Mise au point d'un test ELISA permettant de différencier les animaux vaccinés des animaux infectés par le virus de la maladie d'Aujeszky. J. Rech. Porc., **20,** 141-146.

Eloit, M., Fargeaud, D., Vannier, P. and Toma, B. 1988b. Development of an ELISA test for the differentiation between vaccinated and infected animals by the pseudorabies virus. Vet. Rec., in press.

Mettenleiter, T.C., Lukacs, N. and Rziha, H.J. 1985. Pseudorabies avirulent strains fail to express a major glycoprotein. J. Virol., **56,** 307-311.

Van Oirschot, J.T., Rziha, H.J., Moonen, P.L.J.M., Pol, J.M.A. and Van Zaane, D. 1986. Differentiation of serum antibodies from pigs vaccinated or infected with Aujeszky's disease virus by a competitive enzyme immunoassay. J. Gen. Virol., **67**, 1179-1182.

Van Oirschot, J.T. and De Waal, C.A.H. 1987. An ELISA to distinguish between Aujeszky's disease vaccinated and infected pigs. Vet. Rec., **121**, 305-306.

THE ANTIBODY RESPONSE TO GLYCOPROTEIN I AND THE CONTROL OF AUJESZKY'S DISEASE VIRUS

J.T. van Oirschot

Central Veterinary Institute
PO Box 65, 8200 AB Lelystad, The Netherlands

ABSTRACT

A specific and sensitive ELISA that detects antibodies to 2 epitopes on glycoprotein I (gI) of Aujeszky's disease virus (ADV) is described. This assay enables the distinction of infected pigs and pigs given gI-negative vaccines. For this purpose, serum, whole blood, colostrum or filter paper discs can be used. Infected pigs, whether previously vaccinated or not, develop antibodies to gI that become detectable around 2 weeks post infection and persist for over 1 year. A large herd has probably been freed of ADV by a combination of a continuing vaccination and testing and culling of gI-seropositive pigs. Results of monitoring of a vaccinated herd with the gI-ELISA suggested that elimination of ADV may be achieved without immediate culling of infected pigs.

These results, along with the high efficacy of some gI-negative vaccines, provide a sound basis to implement the "gI-approach" in the control of ADV.

INTRODUCTION

It has been recognized for a long time, that an assay to differentiate between pigs vaccinated or infected with Aujeszky's disease virus (ADV) would be of the utmost importance for the control of ADV. The finding that some vaccine strains of ADV carry deletions in their genomes prompted us to develop such an assay, based on the use of monoclonal antibodies (MAbs)(Van Oirschot *et al.*, 1986). In the present article an improved blocking ELISA is described, together with some results on the antibody response to glycoprotein I (gI) in experimentally or naturally infected pigs.

ELISA TO DETECT ANTIBODIES TO gI

MAbs were prepared and selected for their ability to react with the virulent NIA-3 strain and their inability to react with the avirulent Bartha strain of ADV. Subsequent analyses with radioimmunoprecipitation and Western blot assays showed them to

J. T. van Oirschot (ed.), Vaccination and Control of Aujeszky's Disease, 129–138.

be directed to gI. Two MAbs (MAb 1 and MAb 2) were selected for the gI-ELISA (Van Oirschot *et al.*, 1988). The principle of the gI-ELISA is the blocking of the reaction of 2 MAbs with 2 different epitopes on gI, by antibodies in the test sample (Fig. 1). After determining optimum test conditions the gI-ELISA was done as follows.

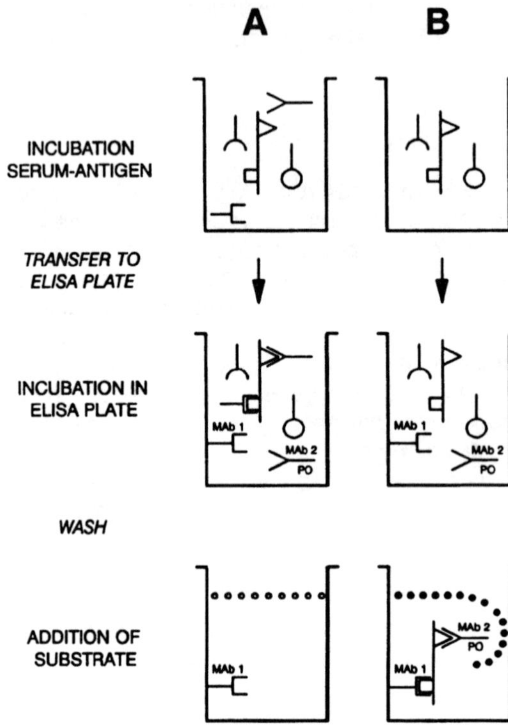

Fig. 1 Schematic diagram of the gI-ELISA. The vertical row under A and B represents serum from an infected pig and a pig vaccinated with a gI- negative vaccine, respectively. Antigen:

1. Polystyrene ELISA microtitre plates were coated by incubation with 100 μl volumes of a 1:5000 dilution of MAb 1 in carbonate buffer, pH 9.5. Incubation was done for 18 hours at 37°C and plates were then stored at 4°C until use.

2. Test sample and antigen were pre-incubated in separate uncoated microtitre plates. For this purpose, 20 μl of test sample was dispensed into wells containing 30 μl of phosphate buffered saline, containing 0.1% bovine serum albumin and 0.05% Tween 80 (PBT). In the case of antibody titration, 2-fold serial dilutions of the test sample in PBT were tested. A 1:10 dilution of antigen in PBT was then added to each well (50 μl per well), and the plates were incubated for 2 hours at 37°C.

Antigen was a freeze-thawed, Nonidet P-40 treated, culture of secondary porcine kidney cells infected with the gI-positive NIA-3 strain of ADV.

3. The ELISA plates were washed 4 times with deionized water containing 0.05% Tween 80 and once with deionized water alone.

4. MAb 2 coupled to horseradish peroxidase was used as conjugate and 30 µl of a 1:500 dilution of the conjugate in PBT was dispensed into all wells of the ELISA plates.

5. The pre-incubated antigen-serum mixtures, in 90 µl volumes, were then transferred from the uncoated plates to the ELISA plates and incubated for 1 hour at 37°C.

6. The plates were washed and 100 µl of substrate solution was added per well. The substrate solution consisted of 0.1 M citrate-phosphate buffer (pH 4), containing 2,2'azinobis(3-ethyl-benzthiazoline-6-sulphonic acid)2NH (0.5 mg/ml) and a 3% solution of freshly added H_2O_2 (2 µl/ml). After 2 hours at room temperature, the plates were read at 405 nm with an automatic ELISA reader.

In each microtitre plate, 4 negative sera and 4 serial 2-fold dilutions of a positive serum were included. The positive serum served as a standard: only those tests were considered valid in which the 2nd or 3rd dilution of the positive serum scored an optical density (OD) value lower than 50% of the mean OD value obtained with the 4 negative control sera. The titre of a serum was expressed as $\log_{10}$ of the reciprocal of the highest serum dilution yielding an OD value of less than 50% of the mean OD value obtained with the 4 negative control sera tested on the same microtitre plate.

The gI-ELISA has been shown to be highly specific, sensitive and reproducible (Van Oirschot *et al.*, 1988). Its sensitivity is evidenced by the detection of antibodies to gI in pigs in which a very limited replication of mild-virulent ADV had taken place. These pigs, which were vaccinated intranasally with a gI-negative vaccine, showed a secondary neutralizing antibody response, but did not show any clinical signs or virus shedding upon contact-challenge (Van Oirschot, 1988). In addition, Fig. 2 shows that the antibody titres to gI are markedly higher than the titres measured in a conventional 1-hour neutralization test, and nearly as high as those measured in a 24-hour neutralization test. Another factor contributing to the sensitivity of the test is that the serum can be tested in a dilution of 1:2. This is in marked contrast with conventional indirect ELISAs where starting dilutions of 1:20 or 1:40 are common.

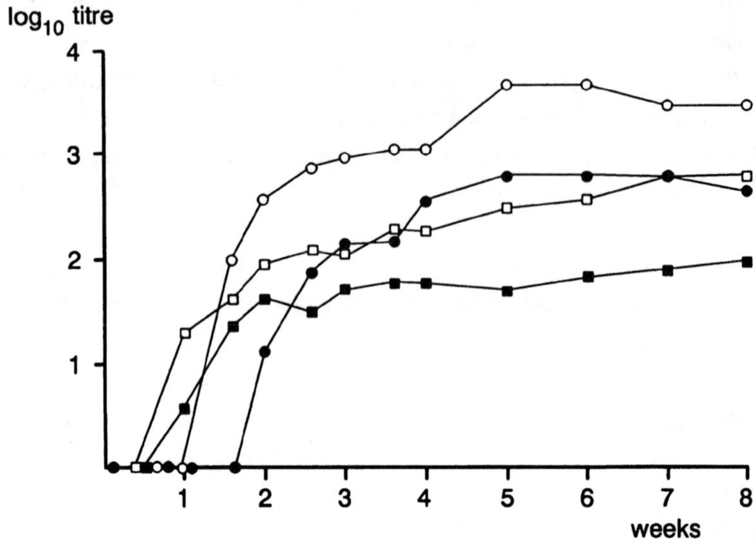

Fig. 2 Antibody development in pigs (n = 4) inoculated with a mildly virulent strain of ADV, measured by conventional "whole virus" ELISA: ○, gI- ELISA: ●, 24-h neutralisation test: □, 1-h neutralisation test: ■.

Apart from serum, plasma, heparinized blood, and filter paper discs containing blood can be used in the gI-ELISA. Table 1 shows the results of a representative experiment in which blood was collected from pigs in the laboratory by various methods at the same time (Table 1). In addition, colostrum or colostral whey can also be examined (data not shown). Additional comparative studies on blood and colostrum collected under field conditions are necessary to determine which method of collection is preferred in the field.

Table 1 OD values obtained by using sera, plasma, heparinized blood samples, and filter paper discs in the gI-ELISA.

Category	Serum	Plasma	Blood	Blood*	Discs
Negative	1615**	1489	1492	1435	1797
Bartha	1807	1661	1582	1479	1496
NIA-3	205	211	185	213	180

*Blood harvested by "vaccinostyle"
**Mean OD values of 2 pigs

LABORATORY EXPERIMENTS

Sera of pigs vaccinated with 1 of 15 vaccines were tested in the gI- ELISA. Six of the vaccine virus strains examined did not induce antibodies to gI: i.e. the Bartha, Begonia, BUK-900, NIA-4, Norden and 783 strain (Gielkens *et al.*, 1988).

After experimental infection of seronegative pigs, gI-antibodies are first detectable approximately 2 weeks post inoculation, whereas neutralizing and ELISA-antibodies appeared 7-10 days post infection. The gI- antibody titre reached a plateau some weeks later and persisted at this level during long periods, perhaps even lifelong (Fig. 2, Table 4).

With regard to combined vaccination-eradication programmes it is of importance that the gI-ELISA also detects pigs which become infected after being vaccinated, because such pigs can harbour latent virus (Van Oirschot and Gielkens, 1984, Wittmann *et al.*, 1984). To examine the antibody development to gI in pigs that were first given gI-negative vaccines and subsequently were challenged with field virus, about 150 post-challenge sera from our ADV serum bank were tested. So far, all pigs that showed a secondary-type neutralizing antibody response after challenge produced antibodies to gI as well. Even pigs that were clinically completely protected against challenge and did not shed virus elicited antibodies to gI. The gI-antibody titres in such pigs were generally lower than in pigs which were seronegative at the time of exposure to a field strain of ADV (Fig. 3, Van Oirschot, 1988).

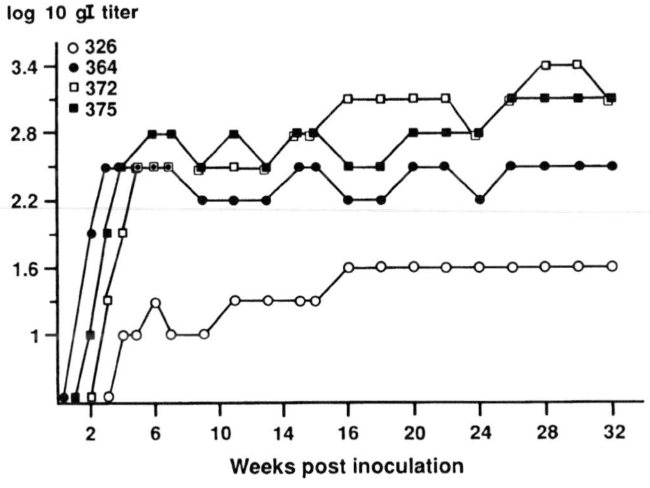

Fig 3 Development and persistence of the gI-antibody response in 3 unvaccinated pigs and 1 vaccinated pig (326) contact-exposed to mildly virulent ADV.

Irrespective whether pigs were previously vaccinated or not, the antibody response to gI in pigs exposed to ADV under experimental conditions, persisted for at least 32 weeks, at which time the experiment ended (Fig. 3, Van Oirschot, 1988).

With regard to distinguishing infected from vaccinated pigs it is important to know whether field viruses that do not induce antibodies to gI circulate among pigs. To shed light on this point, we examined more than 250 isolates from 3 continents and from 14 countries (The Netherlands, Belgium, France, Spain, Italy, Hungary, Federal Republic of Germany, Denmark, Northern Ireland, Ireland, United States of America, Japan, Taiwan, Singapore) for induction of antibodies to gI in pigs and/or *in vitro* gI- expression by immunoperoxidase monolayer assay (Van Oirschot *et al.*, 1986). No gI-negative field viruses have hitherto been found. A bovine ADV isolate exhibiting a defective gI expression (Mettenleiter *et al.*, 1987) also has been found to induce antibodies to gI in pigs (sera were kindly provided by Dr. H.J. Rziha).

Virus isolates are usually recovered from clinical cases of AD. The low-virulent viruses causing subclinical infections are seldom isolated. It is noteworthy, therefore, that we have diagnosed 4 separate subclinical ADV infections among unvaccinated pigs by detecting seroconversion in paired sera by neutralisation test. All 210 pigs involved also had produced antibody to gI. Thus, in 4 cases, less virulent ADV strains had given rise to gI antibody formation. The above results indicate that it is highly unlikely that gI-negative strains of ADV are widespread among the swine population.

FIELD EXPERIMENTS

We have previously reported the probable elimination of ADV from a large multiplyer herd where vaccination with gI-negative vaccines was carried out (Van Oirschot and De Waal, 1987). Vaccination is still continuing and in December 1987, the whole herd was again examined for antibodies to gI. Two sows were found gI-seropositive (Table 2), both had a gI-antibody titre of 20. One sow just had farrowed and its 4-day-old piglets had maternal gI-antibodies, which had waned at 10 weeks of age. Both sows were gI-seronegative in the first rounds of testing. Extensive investigations failed to clarify, how these sows had become gI-seropositive. Introduction of virus into the herd due to the purchase of gilts was not likely, because all incoming stock was quarantined for a month, and only gI-seronegative pigs were admitted to the herd. It also seems unlikely, that these sows were already infected during the first rounds of serological screening, but had no or undetectable levels of gI-antibodies at these times. Reactivation of putative latent virus might then have induced the antibody response against gI. Airborne spread of ADV from neighbouring herds may explain the unexpected finding of the gI-seropositive sows. Anyhow, the infection appeared restricted to only 2 sows. They were culled and the entire herd was again gI-seronegative 2 months later.

Table 2 Results of 6 successive gI-ELISAs in a vaccinated herd, where gI-seropositive pigs were culled.

Date of sampling	Number of gI-seropositives/Numbers of pigs tested Boars	Sows	Gilts	Piglets
27-09-1986	1/3	57/466	0/93	14/177
01-11-1986	0/2	2/436	0/114	9/151
29-11-1986	0/2	0/438	0/88	1/165
16-03-1987	0/2	0/484	0/118	0/152
30-11-1987	0/3	2/522	0/114	0/153
20-02-1988	0/3	0/546	0/79	0/164

Table 3 Number of gI-seropositive breeding pigs in a vaccinated herd during a 1.5 year period.

	Nos. positive/Nos. tested			
	Oct. 86	March 87	Oct. 87	March 88
Boars	1/1	1/2	0/1	0/1
Sows	18/51	14/52	10/59	9/59
Gilts	0/15	0/17	0/8	0/6
Piglets	4/29	7/30	0/21	5/34

Because culling of (pregnant) breeding pigs is a costly operation, the question arose whether immediate culling is essential in order to free a herd of ADV. For this purpose, a vaccinated herd where gI-seropositive pigs were not culled, was monitored for gI-antibody (Van Oirschot and Wijsmuller, 1988). From 1977 the herd was vaccinated with a gI-negative vaccine twice a year; from January 1987 vaccination was done thrice a year. During the 1.5-year monitoring period 1 boar and 4 gilts were purchased. Table 3 shows that from October 1986 to March 1988 the number of gI-seropositive pigs decreased. This was due to removal, by normal turn-over, of old gI-seropositive sows after weaning. Between October 1986 and

March 1987 not any pig became infected. One pig (No 17, Table 3) became gI-seropositive between March and October 1987. In March 1988, 9 pigs were gI-seropositive, 4 of them were already positive in October 1986. Of the remaining 5 pigs, 4 had been purchased in December 1987 and 1 gilt was bred on the farm. The antibodies to gI in the piglets appeared to be maternally derived, because they disappeared with time.

Most sows were replaced by gilts during the 1.5 year observation period. Twenty sows were present during the entire period. Sixteen of them were gI-seronegative and 4 were gI-seropositive, continually. Most of the gI-seropositive pigs had high antibody titres, which persisted at a stable level for 1-1.5 year (Table 4).

Table 4 Antibody titres to gI of the 10 sows that were gI-seropositive in October 1987

Sow No.	Antibody titre in gI-ELISA			
	Oct. 86	March 87	Oct. 87	March 88
17	—	—	20	np
29	160	80	160	80
31	320	320	320	320
32	160	160	160	np
72	320	160	320	160
77	160	160	80	np
111	80	80	80	np
182	320	320	640	np
199	640	320	160	np
200	640	640	640	640

np = not present

The results demonstrate that the continuous presence of a considerable percentage (15-30%) of ADV-infected sows in a thoroughly vaccinated herd did not lead to widespread dissemination of the virus. This suggests that elimination of ADV may be achieved by application of gI-negative vaccines in a strict and intensive vaccination scheme, in conjunction with removal of infected sows at times when it is most economically, e.g. after having weaned their piglets.

CONCLUDING REMARKS

The gI-ELISA is a sensitive and specific test to detect ADV-infected pigs in populations vaccinated with gI-negative vaccines. No gI-negative field strain of ADV has hitherto been found. Field experiences suggest that it is not difficult to eradicate ADV from herds by a programme of continuous vaccination with gI-negative vaccines and testing and immediate culling of gI-seropositive pigs. However, preliminary results suggest that culling of infected pigs may be postponed until times when it is most economically.

Vaccination can greatly reduce the spread of ADV. A number of gI-negative vaccines are commercially available. Some of them belong to the most efficacious ADV vaccines (De Leeuw and Van Oirschot, 1985, Van Oirschot and Gielkens, 1987). The availability of potent gI-negative vaccines and an ELISA to detect antibodies to gI of ADV, which is highly suitable to examine large numbers of samples, opens perspectives for a combined vaccination-eradication program for AD. Such a program would generally comprise 4 phases: intensive vaccination, screening of pigs for antibodies to gI, economic culling of gI-seropositive pigs and eventually abolishment of vaccination.

ACKNOWLEDGEMENTS

The author thanks F. Daus, P.J.L.M. Moonen and H.J. Gerritsen for skilful technical assistance.

REFERENCES

De Leeuw, P.W. and Van Oirschot, J.T. 1985. Vaccines against Aujeszky's disease: evaluation of their efficacy under standardised laboratory conditions. Vet. Quart., 7, 191-197.

Gielkens, A.L.J., Moormann, R.J.M., Van Oirschot, J.T. and Berns, A.J.M. 1988. Vaccine efficacy and innocuity of strain 783 of Aujeszky's disease virus. In: Proc. CEC Seminar "Vaccination and control of Aujeszky's disease". (Ed. J.T. van Oirschot). Brussels, 1988.

Mettenleiter, T.C., Schreurs, C., Thiel, H.J. and Rziha, H.J. 1987. Variability of pseudorabies glycoprotein I expression. Virol., **158**, 141-146.

Van Oirschot, J.T. 1988. Induction of antibodies to gI in pigs exposed to different doses of a mildly virulent strain of Aujeszky's disease virus. Vet. Rec., **122**, 599-603.

Van Oirschot, J.T. and De Waal, C.A.H. 1987. An ELISA to distinguish between Aujeszky's disease vaccinated and infected pigs. Vet. Rec., **121**, 305-306.

Van Oirschot, J.T. and Gielkens, A.L.J. 1984. Intranasal vaccination of pigs against pseudorabies: Absence of vaccinal virus latency and failure to prevent latency of virulent virus. Am. J. Vet. Res., **45**, 2099-2103.

Van Oirschot, J.T. and Gielkens, A.L.J. 1987. Vaccines against Aujeszky's disease: comparison of efficacy, DNA fingerprints and antibody response to glycoprotein I. Vet. Quart., **9**, 37S-49S.

Van Oirschot, J.T., Houwers, D.J., Rziha, H.J. and Moonen, P.J.L.M. 1988. Development of an ELISA to detect antibodies to glycoprotein I of Aujeszky's disease virus: a method for the serological distinction between infected and vaccinated pigs. J. Virol. Meth., in press.

Van Oirschot, J.T., Rziha, H.J., Moonen, P.J.L.M., Pol, J.M.A. and Van Zaane, D. 1986. Differentiation of serum antibodies from pigs vaccinated or infected with Aujeszky's disease virus by a competitive enzyme immunoassay. J. Gen. Virol., **67**, 1179-1182.

Van Oirschot, J.T. and Wijsmuller, J.M. 1988. Monitoring of a vaccinated pig breeding herd for antibody to glycoprotein I of Aujeszky's disease virus. Proc. 10th IPVS Congress, Rio de Janeiro, p. 172.

Wittmann, G., Ohlinger, V. and Rziha, H.J. 1983. Occurrence and reactivation of latent Aujeszky's disease virus following challenge in previously vaccinated pigs. Arch. Virol., **75**, 29-41.

MUCOSAL IMMUNITY OF AUJESZKY'S DISEASE

D. van Zaane, R.A.M. Brouwers, J.T. van Oirschot, J.M.A. Pol, T.G. Kimman

Central Veterinary Institute, Department of Virology
P.O. Box 65, 8200 AB Lelystad, The Netherlands

ABSTRACT

To gain more insight into immunological factors contributing to protection against Aujeszky's disease virus (ADV), we studied the mucosal immune response to this virus in pigs. For this purpose, ELISAs for the detection of ADV-specific porcine IgA, IgM, IgG1, and IgG2 antibodies were developed. ADV-specific IgA and IgM were measured in an antibody capture assay and ADV-specific IgG1 and IgG2 were measured in an indirect double antibody sandwich assay. The assays proved to be sensitive and isotype-specific. After intranasal vaccination of pigs with an attenuated ADV strain predominantly IgM was detected, both in serum and in secretions. After challenge of these pigs with virulent ADV a secondary immune response developed, in which IgG1 and IgG2 were the predominant isotypes in serum and IgA in secretions. The data strongly indicate the existence of mucosal memory in pigs.

INTRODUCTION

Vaccination of pigs against Aujeszky's disease (AD) with modified-live virus or inactivated virus vaccines induces neutralizing antibodies and sensitized lymphocytes in blood and lymphoid organs but confers only partial protection, especially in maternally immune pigs. Systemic immunity seems not to be related to protection (Martin *et al.*, 1986). In laboratory experiments, vaccination by intranasal (IN) route generally results in better protection than vaccination by intramuscular (IM) route, especially in maternally immune pigs (De Leeuw and Van Oirschot, 1985a, Van Oirschot, 1987). These results and the pathogenesis of AD suggest an important role for the mucosal immune system. There have been few studies in this field and knowledge of mucosal immunity in the porcine respiratory tract is limited.

We aim to study the role of the mucosal immune system in protection against AD and to develop methods for an optimal stimulation of mucosal immunity to AD. In this report we describe the development of isotype-specific ELISAs for detection of antibodies against AD virus (ADV) and we present preliminary results with respect to the kinetics of the antibody response after vaccination and infection.

J. T. van Oirschot (ed.), Vaccination and Control of Aujeszky's Disease, 139–149.

MATERIALS AND METHODS

Pigs

Pigs were from the Central Veterinary Institute's "minimal disease" Dutch Landrace herd, which is free of AD. Pigs were born to unvaccinated sows.

Vaccination and challenge

Three SPF pigs (Dutch Landrace, 10-week-old) were IN vaccinated with 10^6 pfu of ADV, strain Bartha. Three months later (98 days post vaccination, dpv) these animals and 2 10-week-old non-vaccinated SPF pigs were IN challenged with 10^5 pfu of ADV, strain NIA-3 as described before (De Leeuw and Van Oirschot, 1985b).

Bodyweight, temperature and clinical signs were recorded from several days before to 10 days after challenge. Virus excretion was determined by titration of saliva samples on secondary porcine kidney cells (De Leeuw *et al.*, 1982).

Sampling procedures

Blood (B), saliva (S), tears (T), faeces (F), lung (L) and nasal (N) secretions were collected regularly. Lung and nasal secretions were collected under anaesthesia (inhalation of N_2O and Halothane®). To collect nasal washings the piglets were fixed horizontally, laying on their back with their nose in a 45° angle down. One nostril was flushed twice with 7 ml of phosphate buffered saline (PBS) containing methylene blue (E_{680} - 1.0) using a 10 ml syringe with rubber adaptor to fit the nostril. Under these conditions no washing fluid was lost in the oropharyngeal cavity. To collect lung fluid the piglets were held in a horizontal position, laying on their abdomen with their head slightly elevated. A catheter (outer diameter = 2.3 mm) was introduced into the main bronchus (using a laryngoscope) until it stucked. Twenty ml of PBS with methylene blue (37°C) was introduced into the lung and 1 minute later it was collected by suction. Tears and saliva were collected using swabs which were extracted with a constant volume of ELISA buffer or tissue culture medium supplemented with 0.1% or 4% calf serum, respectively, to reduce proteolysis. The volume of saliva collected was calculated from the weight difference of the sample recovered after centrifugation of swabs in special containers and the volume of buffer added. This procedure is unfeasible for tears. Faeces was collected and mixed immediately with 4 volumes of ELISA buffer containing 10% calf serum. Dilution factors were calculated from the E_{680}-value of the lavage fluid before and after sampling of lung and nasal secretions. The dilution of faeces was estimated from the weight increase of the sample containers after collection. The dilution of extracted saliva was calculated from the volume of saliva collected and the volume of buffer added. The dilution factor ($\log_{10}$) was 0.4 to 1.3 for saliva, 0.2 to 1.3 for nasal washings and 0.04 to 0.69 for lung washings. Approximately 75% of the samples had dilutions factors differing not more than 0.4. The dilution factor for tears could not be reliably determined but is at least 1.0 ($\log_{10}$).

Reagents for isotype-specific ELISAs

A clarified lysate of secondary pig kidney cells, infected with the NIA-3 strain of ADV, was used as the ADV-antigen preparation. The active fraction of this antigen preparation has a sedimentation coefficient between 10S and 50S, and probably represents a small subviral particle. Each sample was also tested at its starting dilution for non-specific reactions using a clarified lysate of uninfected secondary pig kidney cells instead of the ADV-antigen. Non-specific reactions were not observed with the samples tested.

As capturing or conjugated antibody, a panel of 23 monoclonal antibodies (MCAs) against ADV was tested. The majority of these MCAs react specifically to glycoprotein gI (courtesy to Dr. H.J. Rziha, B.F.A.V., Tübingen) or gII of ADV. MCAs against porcine immunoglobulins were used as isotype-specific reagents (Van Zaane and Hulst, 1987).

ELISAs

ELISAs were generally done as follows. Polystyrene ELISA plates (Dynatech M129A) were coated with antigen or antibodies in 50 mM $NaHCO_3$, pH 9.6, or PBS, pH 7.4, for 16 h at 37°C. All other reagents except the substrate were diluted in ELISA buffer (0.5 M NaCl, 10 mM PO_4 (3-), pH 7.2, 0.05% w/v Tween 80) and were added in predetermined optimal concentration in a volume of 100 μl. Sample dilutions and conjugate solutions contained 1% ovalbumin to reduce the background staining. Following each incubation step, plates were washed 10 times with 0.05% w/v Tween 80 in tap-water, using a home-made ELISA plate washing device. As the final step in all ELISAs ABTS was used as substrate. Absorbance was measured using a Titertek Multiskan at 450 nm. The reciprocal of the highest dilution of a test sample yielding an E_{405} 0.300 was taken as titer.

RESULTS

Development of isotype-specific ELISAs

Based on our experience with isotype-specific ELISAs for bovine rotavirus antibodies and bovine respiratory syncytial virus antibodies (Van Zaane and

IJzerman, 1984; Kimman *et al.*, 1987) similar assays were developed for the detection of IgG1, IgG2, IgM and IgA antibodies against ADV in swine. An indirect double antibody sandwich (IDAS) assay appeared optimal for the detection of IgG1 and IgG2 antibodies, whereas for the detection of IgM and IgA an antibody capture assay (ACA) appeared to be the test of choice. The principles of the assays are schematically shown in Fig. 1.

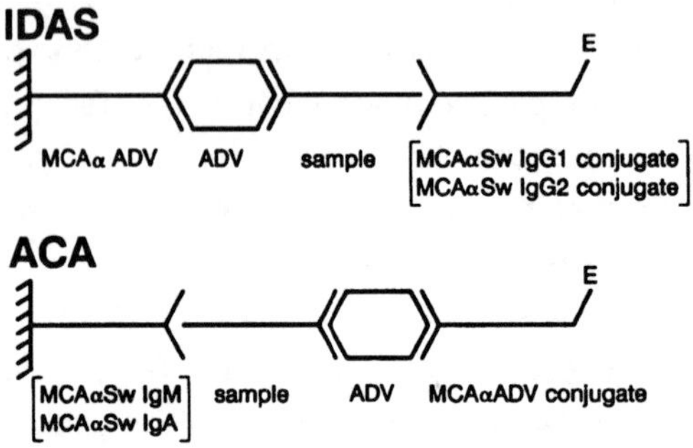

Fig. 1 Isotype-specific ELISAs for ADV antibodies. IDAS: Indirect double antibody sandwich assay; ACA: Antibody capture assay; MCA: Monoclonal antibody; ADV: Aujeszky's disease virus.

After the selection of optimal reagents and assay conditions, highly specific and sensitive assays were developed. Since the use of polyclonal antisera against ADV in the IDAS and the ACA resulted in high backgrounds, a panel of 23 MCAs against ADV was tested for their performance as capturing or conjugated antibodies. Four MCAs (45.11.1a, 45.16.4b, 45.19.1a and 45.21.2b) appeared to be highly effective as capturing antibody in the IDAS, whereas 3 other MCAs (45.24.1a, 45.24.4a and 45.25.2a) were found to be optimal as conjugate in the ACA. These MCAs reacted specifically to glycoprotein gII. Characteristics of the MCAs against the porcine immunoglobulins are given in Table 1. The protocol and reagents finally used are summarized concisely in Table 2.

The isotype specificity of the IDAS-G1, IDAS-G2, ACA-M AND ACA-A was analyzed using samples which were negative for one or more isotypes (Table 3). These results show that all assays detect only its homologous isotype (titer difference at least 2.8 $\log_{10}$ units, except for the difference in IgG1 and IgG2 titer of sample 3B13). The sensitivity of the isotype-specific ELISAs was compared to that of a neutralization assay (De Leeuw *et al.*, 1982) using a 24 hr incubation period of the antibody-virus mixture (Table 4). In general, the ELISAs appeared to be more sensitive.

TABLE 1 Isotype-specific MCAs used in the IDAS and ACA

MCA	Mouse Ig-isotype	titer (a) against porcine Ig-specificity G1	G2	M	A	
23.49.2	G1	6	—	—	—	IgG1
34.2.1a	G1	3	6	—	2	IgG2
28.4.1	G1	—	—	5	(4)b	IgM
27.9.1	G1	—	—	—	6	IgA

a) titer in an indirect ELISA expressed as $\log_{10}$
b) shallow titration curve with low E_{450} at high MCA concentration

TABLE 2 Protocol and reagents for isotype-specific ADV ELISAs

Step	IDAS-G1	IDAS-G2	ACA-M	ACA-A	Incubation
Coating	45.11.1a	45.11.1a	28.4.1	27.9.1	overnight at 37°C
Antigen	ADV (NIA-3) or control cell lysate				1 hr at 37C
Sample	serum/saliva/tears/lung secretion/nasal secretion/faeces				1 hr at 37C
Conjugate	23.49.2	34.2.1a	45.24.1a	45.24.1a	1 hr at 37C
Substrate	ABTS	ABTS	ABTS	ABTS	room temperature

Coating buffer for the IDAS was 50 mM $NaHCO_3$, pH 9.6; for the ACA PBS was used. The starting dilution for serum and faeces was 1/20, for the other samples 1/5.

TABLE 3 Isotype specificity of ADV ELISAs

Sample	IDAS-G1	IDAS-G2	ACA-M	ACA-A
1B132	4.6(a)	4.2	—(b)	—
3B13	2.3	—	4.0	—
2B10	—	—	4.5	—
6L106	—	—	>4.6	—
3T115	—	—	—	3.4
3T118	—	—	—	3.6

a) expressed as $\log_{10}$ titer
b) — : < 1.1 for B-samples; < 0.5 for L- and T-samples;
B = serum, L = lung fluid, T = tears.

TABLE 4 Comparison of antibody titers in isotype-specific ADV ELISAs and neutralization assay

Sample	Neutralization	IDAS-G1	IDAS-G2	ACA-M	ACA-A
Ref	2.7 (a)	3.7	3.4	nt	nt
6B111	3.7	4.2	3.5	>4.6	—
4B111	3.6	4.0	4.0	3.2	3.2
1L111	0.6	—	—	—	1.2
3L111	1.7	1.5	—	—	3.6
4L111	0.5	—	—	—	2.1
1T111	0.6	—	—	—	2.1
3T111	0.9	—	—	—	2.9
4T111	0.9	—	—	0.7	2.6

a) expressed as $\log_{10}$ titer; B = serum, L = lung fluid, T = tears

Responses to intranasal vaccination and challenge

The clinical and virological data of this experiment are summarized in Fig. 2. The vaccinated pigs appeared to be well protected against intranasal challenge with virulent ADV. One animal (no. 1) showed growth retardation of 5 days compared to 16 days for the control animal; the second control animal died at 8 days postchallenge. Animal no. 1 was also the only one which had fever (1 day). Animals nos. 3 and 4 developed no clinical signs. Virus was present in the saliva of vaccinated pigs nos. 1 and 3, but at a lower level and for a shorter period as compared to the control pigs nos. 5 and 6. In the saliva of vaccinated animal no. 4 no virus was detectable.

A detailed analysis of the isotype-specific immune response to ADV in serum and tears of 1 animal (no. 3) is shown in Fig. 3. Responses in other secretions were largely the same as in tears. Other pigs reacted largely similar. The response after vaccination is characterized by the almost simultaneous appearance at about 8 dpv of IgM anti-ADV antibodies in both serum and secretions, except faeces. Later, in serum IgG1 (10-13 dpv) and IgG2 (13-20 dpv) and in some animals also IgA antibodies were detected. In secretions, the IgM antibody response was followed by a weak or moderate IgA antibody response from 10-13 dpv onwards, but no IgG1 or IgG2 antibodies were detectable. IgA antibodies were not consistently present in all secretions.

Upon challenge, strong and rapid IgG1, IgG2 and IgA responses were observed in serum. IgG1 and IgG2 persisted at high levels till at least 3 months after challenge, whereas the titer of the IgA antibodies fell gradually to a lower level. However, IgA antibody activity was still detectable at the end of the experiment in 2 out of 3 animals. In secretions, IgA antibody was the predominant isotype, although other isotypes were usually detectable in low titers and intermittently.

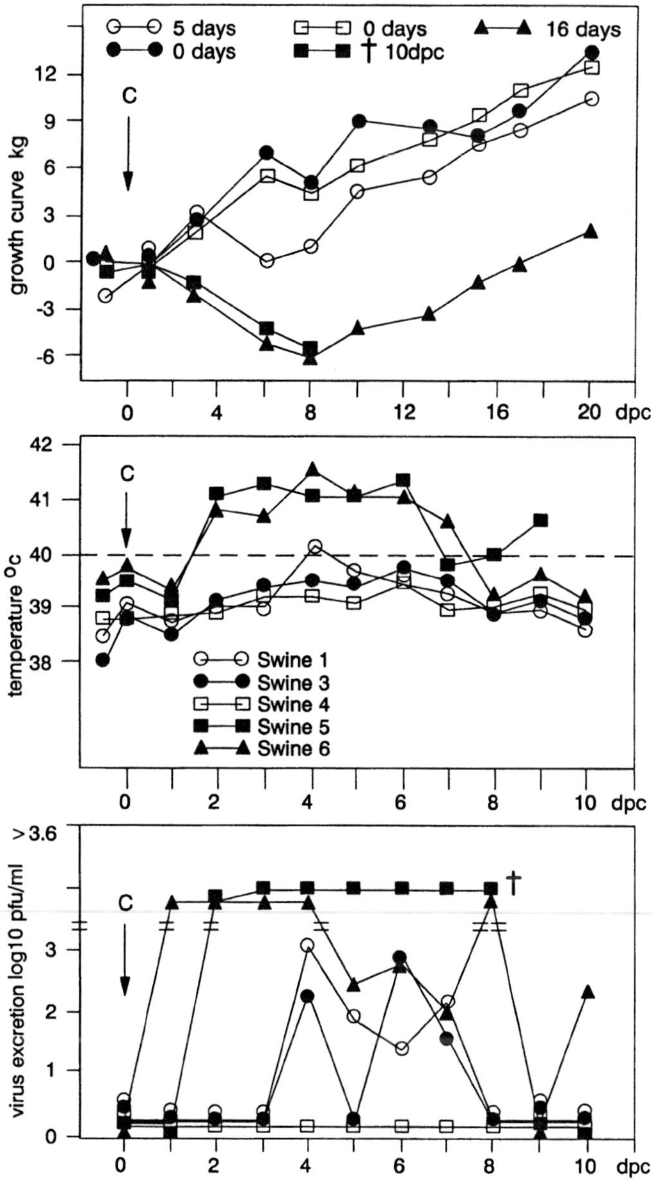

Fig. 2 Clinical and virological data from the vaccination experiment. Pigs nos. 1, 3 and 4 were vaccinated intranasally with ADV strain Bartha, and challenged intranasally with ADV strain NIA-3 at 98 days after vaccination. Control pigs nos. 5 and 6 were challenged only.

The antibody response of a non-vaccinated animal after challenge was similar to that after intranasal vaccination. However, IgM and IgA were detected earlier in serum and secretions and their titers were usually higher.

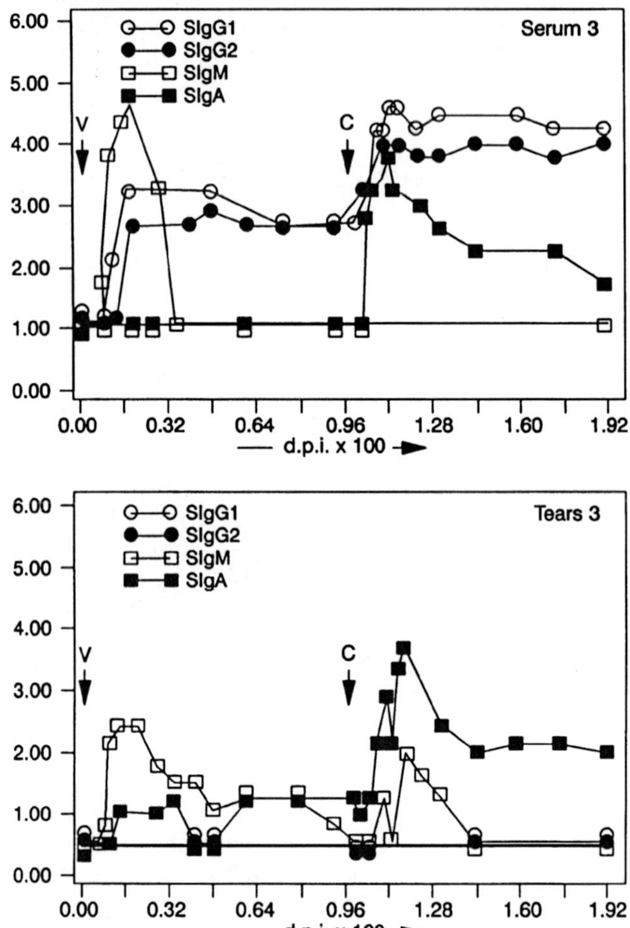

Fig. 3 Isotype-specific immune response to ADV in serum and tears of pig no. 3 after intranasal vaccination and challenge with ADV. Titers are expressed as $\log_{10}$. See also legend to Fig. 2.

DISCUSSION

ELISAs are very suitable for the isotype-specific analysis of antibody activity in large numbers of samples (Van Zaane and IJzerman, 1984; Kimman *et al.*, 1987). For the detection of ADV-specific IgA and IgM ACAs were used. The advantages of the ACA are that: 1) competition between isotypes (inter-isotype competition) does not occur; 2) non-specific reactions are generally infrequent; and 3) interference by rheumatoid factors is highly unlikely (Van Zaane and IJzerman, 1984). However, this assay appeared not to be suitable for the detection of IgG1 and IgG2 antibodies due to competition effects within an isotype (intra-isotype competition). Therefore, for detection of ADV-specific IgG1 and IgG2 IDAS assays were developed. These 4 ELISAs appeared to be isotype-specific, sensitive and thus useful for the study of the local and systemic immune response to ADV. It should be noted here that the absolute sensitivity of the various isotype-specific ELISAs might be different. This is difficult to assess but might interfere with a reliable comparison of titers of different antibody isotypes.

The first data obtained show that both the systemic and the mucosal primary immune response after intranasal vaccination or infection with ADV is characterized by the production and/or secretion of IgM antibodies. During the secondary systemic immune response, IgG1 and IgG2 antibodies were the predominant isotypes, accompanied by IgA antibodies at lower levels. In secretions, IgA is the main antibody isotype detected in secondary responses. These data also indicate the existence of mucosal memory in pigs.

Fig. 4 shows a comparison of the IgA antibody responses in serum and lung wash fluid of vaccinated pigs and a control animal after challenge. It seems that the animals with the weakest IgA response were less well protected than animals with a strong IgA memory response in serum and secretions. This might suggest a role for the humoral mucosal immune system in protection in AD after intranasal vaccination. Whether this is a significant correlation will be the subject of further study.

Using the techniques described in this paper, our present research is directed at the immune response after experimental infection and reinfection with ADV strain NIA-3 and the immune response after intramuscular vaccination with inactivated vaccine and challenge with ADV-NIA-3. Subsequently, the influence of maternal antibodies on the development of mucosal immunity after vaccination and infection will be studied.

ACKNOWLEDGEMENTS

This work was supported by CEC-contract no. 3910. We thank Dr. L.A.M.G. van Leengoed for introducing to us the lung lavage technique.

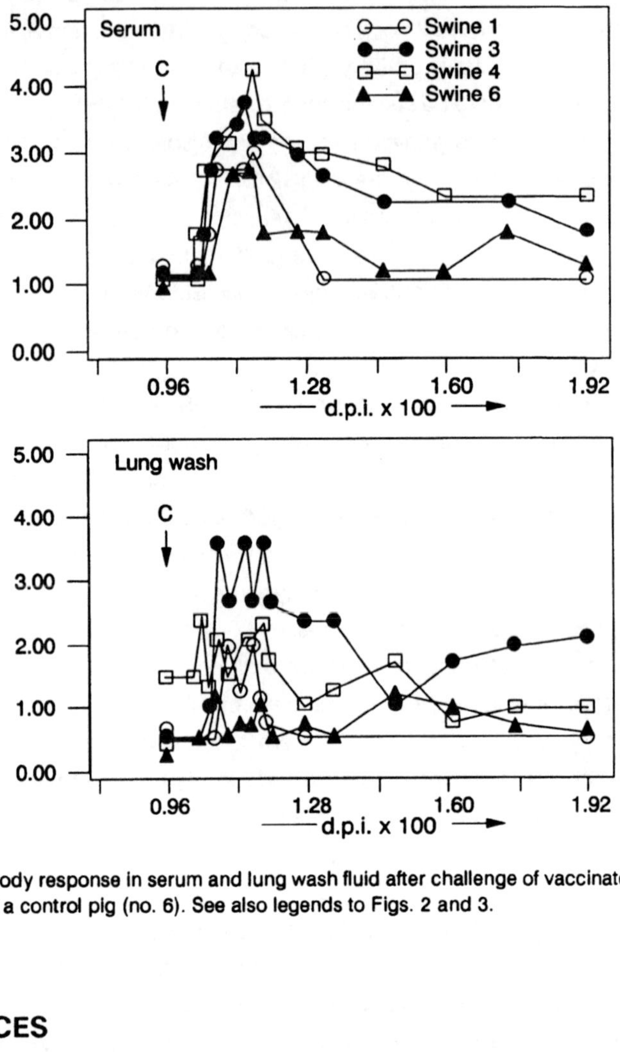

Fig. 4 IgA antibody response in serum and lung wash fluid after challenge of vaccinated pigs (nos. 1, 3 and 4) and a control pig (no. 6). See also legends to Figs. 2 and 3.

REFERENCES

De Leeuw, P.W., Wijsmuller, J.M., Zantinga, J.W. and Tielen, M.J.M. 1982. Intranasal vaccination of pigs against Aujeszky's disease. 1. Comparison of intranasal or parenteral vaccination with an attenuated vaccine in 12 week old pigs from immunized dams. Vet. Quarterly, **4**, 49-56.

De Leeuw, P.W. and Van Oirschot, J.T. 1985a. Intranasal vaccination of pigs against Aujeszky's disease: comparison with inactivated vaccines in pigs with low maternal antibody titers. Res. Vet. Sci., **39**, 34-38.

De Leeuw, P.W. and Van Oirschot, J.T. 1985b. Vaccines against Aujeszky's disease: evaluation of their efficacy under standardized laboratory conditions. Vet. Quarterly, **7**, 191-197.

Kimman, T.G., Westenbrink, F., Straver, P.J. and Van Zaane, D. 1987. Isotype-specific ELISAs for the detection of antibodies to bovine respiratory syncytial virus. Res. Vet. Sci., **43,** 180-187.

Martin, S., Wardley, R.C. and Donaldson, A.J. 1986. Functional antibody responses in pigs vaccinated with live and inactivated Aujeszky's disease virus. Res. Vet. Sci., **41,** 331-335.

Van Oirschot, J.T. 1987. Intranasal vaccination of pigs against Aujeszky's disease: comparison with one or two doses of attenuated vaccines in pigs with high maternal antibody titres. Res. Vet. Sci., **42,** 12-16.

Van Zaane, D. and IJzerman, J. 1984. Monoclonal antibodies against bovine immunoglobulins and their use in isotype-specific ELISAs for rotavirus antibody. J. Immunol. Meth., **72,** 427-441.

Van Zaane, D. and Hulst, M.M. 1987. Monoclonal antibodies against porcine immunoglobulin isotypes. Vet. Immunol. and Immunopathol., **16,** 23-36.

QUALITY CONTROL OF THE SEROLOGICAL DIAGNOSIS OF AUJESZKY'S DISEASE IN FRANCE

B.Toma, M. Eloit

Laboratoire National de Référence de la maladie d'Aujeszky
Ecole Nationale Vétérinaire d'Alfort
94704 Maisons-Alfort Cedex France

ABSTRACT

During last years a quality control has been applied, to 1) ELISA kits to be commercialized, and 2) laboratories approved to perform serological tests on Aujeszky's disease. The percentage of unsatisfactory quality control results produced by approved laboratories has gradually decreased: 24% in 1984, 7% in 1985, 4% in 1986 and 0% in 1988. These good results partly agree with the quality control results of batches of ELISA kits.

The protocol of quality control of ELISA kits used in France is presented. Until now it has been used only for conventional ELISA kits. In the future, it will be used also for kits which allow distinction between infected pigs and pigs vaccinated with gI deleted strains. It seems necessary to develop this kind of control in the European Community and to harmonize the protocols of quality control between the countries of the European Community.

INTRODUCTION

The control of Aujeszky's disease (AD) usually includes a systematic serological screening of pig sera for antibodies to AD virus (ADV). Hundreds of thousands of sera must, therefore, be tested each year. For the international trade of pigs, the quality of the serological tests is very important. Consequently, it is necessary to use serological tests with a very good sensitivity and an excellent specificity. During the last years, ELISAs has been used more and more to screen pigs for AD. Commercial kits became available and now many laboratories can use them routinely.

The quality of the commercialized kits will largely determine the quality of the results produced by the laboratories using the kits. Therefore, in France a quality control is employed on 1) each batch of commercialized ELISA kits, and 2) on the laboratories doing the serological diagnosis of AD.

Previously, studies have been done (Toma and Benet, 1982), on a national and European level, to define an international reference serum, which is a weakly

J. T. van Oirschot (ed.), Vaccination and Control of Aujeszky's Disease, 151–158.

positive serum, that must be found positive in all cases in all laboratories. This serum is available since several years and is used as a reference for the preparation of the quality controls conducted in France.

In this paper, we present the French experience of quality control in the serological diagnosis of AD; an experience that could be used as a basis of reflection on harmonization of a protocol in the European Community (EC).

QUALITY CONTROL OF ELISA KITS

This control began in March 1984 and has been organized around the international reference serum.

Protocol

In the beginning there were no methods for the distinction of infected pigs and pigs vaccinated with a deleted strain. New modalities have recently been introduced for the control of kits able to do this distinction, and which begin to be proposed for commercialization. We will give, below, the actual protocol.

1. Conditions before the control.

1.1. Reagents.

A kit must include all the reagents necessary for the study of samples. Only will be admitted diluting reagents in a buffer, which must be furnished in a state ready for use or in a concentrated form. Any preparation of reagents with material not available in the kit must be excluded. All the reagents of a batch will receive an identification reference used only for this batch. Any modification of one of the biological reagents (antigen, sera, monoclonal antibodies, conjugate...) will implicate a new control with a different reference. The indications on the notice must be in French. This notice must give all the information about the steps of the reaction and the criteria for the interpretation of the results. It must also indicate whether the kit can be used with samples of blood dried on paper discs (individually or together) and the protocol to test this kind of samples.

1.2. Expedition to the laboratory.

At least 6 plates of each batch and all necessary reagents must be sent to the reference laboratory. Together with these reagents must be sent all the information about the results got by the producer during the control of the corresponding batch.

2. Control protocol.

2.1. Sera

2.1.1. Sera for both classical kits and kits for the differentiation of infected from vaccinated pigs.

- Sera from healthy pigs (Nos. 1 to 4).
- A serum from a healthy pig, vaccinated several times against parvovirosis. This serum can give a high level of non-specific background with some batches (No. 5).
- A serum with the same level of antibodies as the international reference serum (No. 6).
- The same serum diluted 1:2 (No. 7).
- Four dilutions of a positive serum in a negative serum (undiluted, 1:4, 1:16, 1:64). The 1:16 dilution has an antibody titer similar to that of the international reference serum (Nos. 8, 9, 10 and 11).
- Three sera from infected pigs (Nos. 12, 13 and 14).

2.1.2. Specific sera for kits enabling distinction between infected and vaccinated pigs.

Ten sera of pigs vaccinated with the Bartha strain (Nos. 15 to 24).

2.2. Protocol

2.2.1. Initial control

2.2.1.1. Classical kits. Three plates are tested. Each serum (Nos. 1 to 14) is tested 3 times in each plate.

2.2.1.2. Kits for differentiation. Three plates are tested. Each serum (Nos. 1 to 14) is tested 3 times in 2 plates. The 10 sera (Nos. 15 to 24) are tested 3 times in a plate.

2.2.2. Additional controls. One plate is tested half-way the validity period and another at the end of this period.

2.2.2.1. Classical kits. The sera Nos. 1 to 14 are tested 3 times in the plate.

2.2.2.2. Kits for differentiation. The sera Nos. 1 to 14 are tested twice in the plate. The sera 15 to 24 are tested once in the plate.

2.3 Studied parameters.

2.3.1. Specificity. $\frac{\text{Number of sera found negative among the negative sera}}{\text{Number of negative sera}}$

Negative sera are Nos. 1 to 5 for classical kits and Nos. 1 to 5 and 15 to 24 for kits for differentiation.

2.3.2. Sensitivity. $\dfrac{\text{Number of sera found positive among the positive sera}}{\text{Number of positive sera}}$

Sera considered as positive are all sera with a level of antibodies equal or higher than that of the international reference serum (Nos. 6, 8, 9, 10, 12, 13, 14).

2.3.3. Variation index of weakly positive sera (Nos. 6, 7, 10, 11).

2.3.4. Variation index of positive sera (Nos. 8, 9, 12, 13, 14).

These 2 indexes are calculated by variance analysis for the initial control.

2.3.5. Dosis-effect law. It is studied from the curve of responses observed with the 4 dilutions of a positive serum (Nos. 8 to 11).

2.4. Results.

The kits are approved for commercialization in France at the end of the initial control if: the specificity and sensitivity index = 1, and the variation indexes and dosis-effect law are satisfactory. For the additional controls the same criteria are used. If the results of the quality control are not good, the producer is informed and the kit must be taken off the market.

General results

Table 1 shows that some companies have proposed only satisfactory batches, whereas others have presented batches which were not approved or have been taken off the market after the additional controls. It also shows that, generally, the results were better during the last 2 years than in the beginning.

Table 1 General results of quality controls of ELISA kits proposed to be commercialized in France from 1984.

Year	Company				
	A	B	C	D	E
1984	S 5*	S 2	NS 2		
		NS 1**			
1985	S 3	NS 1	S 2		
		NS 1	NS 1		
1986	S 6	S 2			
1987	S 3	S 2		S 7	
1988-june	S 3		S 2	S 7	S 1

* 5 batches of ELISA kits which are considered satisfactory (= S).

** 1 batch of ELISA kits which is considered non-satisfactory (= NS), some batches were found non-satisfactory after 3-5 months of storage.

Discussion

The quality control used in France does not provide an absolute guarantee for the absence of difficulties and errors during the routine use of the approved batches of ELISA kits. First, the stability of reagents is not tested in the initial control, and therefore additional controls are done during the validity period of each batch. Second, the number of sera used for the control is low, especially for negative sera, and these sera can not cover all risks of non-specificity. Therefore, a batch of a company having scored good results at the initial control, with only a background somewhat higher than that of previous batches, may lead to difficulties in the field. For example, sera from a seronegative pig might then be considered weakly positive. However, we take the line that the protocol of quality control is able to identify the main problems of sensitivity and specificity of kits proposed for commercialization.

The results of the initial quality control must be carefully studied, because kits with are just marginally satisfactory, may pose problems when used for testing field sera. The responsability of the director of the reference laboratory can be high and his task is a delicate one. In case of disagreement about the commercialization of a batch, the criteria used for the negative decision must be strong enough not to be contested. The economic consequences may be profound. On the other hand, in case of approving a batch which gives problems in the field, the quality of the control by the reference laboratory may be questioned.

Companies market their ELISA kits in several EC countries. In the absence of quality control in some countries or in the case of using different protocols we take the risk that the same batch could be approved in one EC country and not in another. The harmonization of protocols for quality control in different EC countries is therefore recommended.

QUALITY CONTROL OF DIAGNOSTIC LABORATORIES

When the epidemiological studies on AD in France began, the number of diagnostic laboratories strongly increased. From 1979 to 1982, 5 studies have been done on check test sera, in the beginning only French laboratories participated, later some European laboratories became involved. The quality control of the approved laboratories began in 1984.

Protocol

The group of studied sera is composed of sera from AD free and unvaccinated pigs, sera from infected or vaccinated animals and sera with antibody titers comparable to the titer of the EC reference serum (several dilutions) (Table 2). Each serum is presented once, or more often 2 to 4 times. The quantity of the sera is limited, so that the laboratories can test them only 2 or 3 times. The results must be available not later than 1 month after the arrival of the sera at the laboratory.

Table 2 Origin of the sera for the 1986 quality control and results of the approved laboratories.

No. serum	Number of samples	Origin	Results ELISA	VNT
1	3	—	46/47*	8/8
2	3	—	44/45	6/6
3	3	—	48/48	8/8
4	3	—	47/48	9/9
5	3	—	47/47	9/9
6	3	—	48/48	9/9
7	3	+ **	48/48	8/9
8	2	+	42/48	8/9
9	2	+	17/48	5/9
10	1	+	3/48	1/9
11	2	+	48/48	9/9
12	2	+	48/48	9/9
13	2	+	48/48	9/9

*Numerator: number of laboratories with negative (Nos. 1 to 6) or positive (Nos. 7 to 13) results, Denominator: number of laboratories performing the test.
** Serum No. 7 has a titer in the ELISA equal to the EC reference serum, sera Nos. 8, 9 and 10 are a 1:2, 1:4 and 1:8 dilution of serum No. 7.

The sera are sent to the laboratories as sera for quality control, but once they were sent as if they were field samples. The reference of each serum differs from one laboratory to another to avoid exchange of results between laboratories. In 1988, for the first time, some blood samples were presented dried on paper discs and these had to be studied separately or after mixing. For the interpretation of the results, all the sera with an antibody titer higher than that of the EC reference serum had to be considered positive. For the sera with a lower titer than that of the EC reference serum, the results "positive", "negative" or "doubtful" were accepted. For the sera without ADV-antibodies only the result "negative" was accepted. We, generally, considered a result as satisfactory if the right answer was given for all the samples of the same sera.

Results

The number of laboratories participating in this quality control increased from 1984 to 1988. The proportion of laboratories with good results has increased as well (Table 3).

Table 3 General results of quality control of the approved laboratories from 1984 to 1988.

Year	Number of laboratories	
	participating	with good results
1984	29	22 (76%)
1985	41	38 (93%)
1986	50	48 (96%)
1988	55	55 (100%)

In 1984, the mistakes of the 7 laboratories with non satisfactory results came from errors in sensitivity or specificity or both. In 1985 and 1986, only errors in specificity have been recorded. In 1988, the results produced with blood collected on paper discs were also satisfactory. The details of the results in 1986 are presented in Table 2.

Discussion

Table 3 shows an increase in the number of laboratories that performed well. This amelioration is due, on one side, to the increasing experience in ELISA testing of these laboratories, and on the other side, to the increasing quality of the commercialized ELISA kits.

The quality of serological diagnosis of AD in a country depends on the quality of: 1) the companies producing the kits, 2) the approved diagnostic laboratories, and 3) the reference laboratory. The quality of the companies and of the approved laboratories must be evaluated by the reference laboratory. The quality of the reference laboratory must be guaranteed by cooperation between reference laboratories in several countries. Therefore, for the quality control of the serological diagnosis of AD international cooperation is necessary.

ACKNOWLEDGEMENTS

We thank Miss M. Andriamanga and A. Fournier for their excellent technical collaboration.

REFERENCES

Toma, B. and Benet, J.J. 1982. Méthodologie de l'harmonisation de la sérologie de la maladie d'Aujeszky. Epidemiologie et santé animale, **2**, 42-55.

SUMMARY

Ben-Porat *et al.* showed that gI, gII and gIII are equally expressed on the surface of infected cells. They had experimental evidence that in mice gIII induced more cytotoxic T lymphocytes than gI, and that gIII contributed to a larger extent to the pool of neutralizing antibody in pig serum than gI. In addition, they showed that mice inoculated with TK^-/$gIII^-$ deletion mutants were less well protected against challenge than TK^- mutants with deletions either in gX or gI.

Eloit *et al.* developed competitive ELISAs for detection of antibodies against gI and gIII. Pigs vaccinated with Bartha or BUK strains did not develop antibodies to gI, whereas they did produce antibodies to gIII. Maternally derived antibodies can persist for about 5 months. They further showed that both tests were suitable to perform epidemiological surveys in the field.

Van Oirschot developed an ELISA that detects antibodies to 2 different epitopes on gI. An indication of its sensitivity is that it detects antibodies to gI in pigs with a very low level of virus replication. The antibody response to gI persisted for more than a year, and probably persists even lifelong. Field experiments suggest that it can be easy to eliminate ADV from a vaccinated herd by testing and culling procedures. Perhaps, culling can take place at times when it is most economically.

Kimman *et al.* described the development of isotype-specific ELISAs for measuring antibodies to ADV, for the study of mucosal immunity. After intranasal vaccination or infection, IgM was the predominant isotype in both serum and secretions. After challenge, IgG1 and IgG2 were predominantly present in serum and IgA in secretions. These results are evidence for the existence of mucosal memory. No correlation has yet been established between IgA responses in secretions and protection against infection.

Toma and Eloit described procedures currently used in France for the quality control of ELISA kits. Each batch of kits must be controlled before commercialization. During recent years most batches of commercial ELISA kits were found to be of good quality. In the future it will be also necessary to perform quality control on ELISA kits for differentiation of infected or vaccinated pigs. The laboratories in France examine a number of sera, and they must get good results to be officially approved for performing ELISAs. An international harmonization of quality control of kits is proposed.

J. T. van Oirschot (ed.), Vaccination and Control of Aujeszky's Disease, 159.

4. EPIDEMIOLOGY AND CONTROL OF AUJESZKY'S DISEASE

Chairpersons M.B. Pensaert and D.G. Thawley

AUJESZKY'S DISEASE VIRUS REPLICATION IN TONSILS AND RESPIRATORY TRACT OF NON-IMMUNE AND IMMUNE PIGS

C. Miry, M.B. Pensaert

Laboratory of Virology, Faculty of Veterinary Medicine, State University of Gent, Casinoplein 24, 9000 Gent, Belgium

ABSTRACT

The aim of the present work was to compare the sites and the extent of virulent Aujeszky's disease virus replication in tonsils and respiratory tract of non-immune pigs and in pigs immune after previous experimental infection (with virulent virus) or vaccination (with an inactivated parenterally or attenuated vaccine intranasally administered).

Virus replication in tonsils and respiratory tract in non-immune pigs was followed both after oronasal and after intratracheal inoculation. Immune pigs were challenged by a combined oronasal/intratracheal inoculation.

Oronasal inoculation of non-immune pigs resulted in virus replication which was extensive in tonsils and upper respiratory tract, but remained limited to scarce foci of infected cells in the lungs. Upon intratracheal inoculation, however, virus replication started in the deeper airways (terminal bronchioli, alveolar cells, interstitial cells and alveolar macrophages), and spread towards bronchioli and bronchi. The infection took place in the total lung and all cell types were involved. Infection of free bronchio-alveolar cells was consistently found.

In tonsils and nasal mucosa of pigs immune after infection, replication of challenge virus was totally prevented. This was not the case in pigs immune after vaccination. Titers were markedly reduced in pigs vaccinated with the inactivated vaccine but not in those with the attenuated vaccine.

In the lungs, neither infection-immunity nor vaccination-immunity was able to prevent infection upon challenge. Replication of challenge virus was drastically reduced in infection-immune pigs, whereas little reduction was noted in intranasally vaccinated pigs. A considerable reduction was seen in pigs vaccinated with inactivated vaccine.

In all the immune animals, free bronchio-alveolar cells and cells in the alveoli were most consistently involved in the infection process.

INTRODUCTION

Primary target sites of Aujeszky's disease virus (ADV) in feeder pigs upon experimental inoculation were shown to be the nasopharyngeal, tracheal and pulmonary regions, as virus was isolated from these organs (Wittmann *et al.*, 1980). Even though virus morphogenesis was demonstrated in cells of the lung

J. T. van Oirschot (ed.), Vaccination and Control of Aujeszky's Disease, 163–173.

(Baskerville, 1973), the pathogenesis of ADV infection in the lower respiratory tract still remains unclear. More data on the sites or cell types involved may explain why and where virus replication still can occur in immune pigs. Indeed, even though vaccination reduces clinical disease and economic losses (Pensaert and Maes, 1984), it fails to prevent infection and virus replication at the primary sites (Wittmann *et al.*, 1982). Pigs vaccinated with inactivated or attenuated vaccines still can excrete virus in reduced quantities in nasal or oropharyngeal secretions upon challenge (McFerran *et al.*, 1979; Donaldson *et al.*, 1984; De Leeuw and Van Oirschot, 1985; Van Oirschot and Gielkens, 1987).

The question can be asked which cell types can become infected with ADV independently of the immune status of the animal. It was the aim of the present work to study the sites and the extent of virus replication in tonsils and respiratory tract in non-immune pigs, and comparison was made with virus replication occurring in pigs, immune after infection or after vaccination.

MATERIALS AND METHODS

Experimental design

In this study, 3 groups of pigs (designated A, B and C) were used at 10 weeks of age. At the start of the experiments, all pigs were negative for ADV antibodies using a standard serum neutralization test (Andries *et al.*, 1978). The virus used for inoculations or challenge procedures consisted of a virulent field strain 75V19 of ADV (Andries *et al.*, 1978).

In group A (non-immune pigs), 4 pigs were inoculated oronasally (ON) with $10^5 TCID_{50}$ in 5 ml inoculum and euthanized 3, 4, 5 and 7 days post inoculation, respectively. Five additional pigs were inoculated intratracheally (IT). Intratracheal inoculation was performed as described previously (Maes *et al.*, 1984) with $10^{7.5} TCID_{50}$ virulent ADV in 8 ml inoculum and the pigs were euthanized 0.5, 1 or 2 days post inoculation, respectively, as described in Table 1.

Group B (immune after infection) consisted of 9 pigs which were inoculated ON with $10^5 TCID_{50}$ in 5 ml inoculum. The pigs were allowed to recover and challenged 1 or 2 months later.

Group C (immune after vaccination) consisted of 9 pigs which were vaccinated. Four pigs were vaccinated twice, with 2 weeks interval, with an inactivated vaccine (Nobivac®) and 5 pigs were vaccinated intranasally with an attenuated vaccine(Suvaxyn I.N.®). They were challenged 1 month after the last vaccination.

Four weeks after infection or vaccination, blood samples were collected from all the pigs of group B and C. Additionally, lung lavage was done at that time on 4 pigs of group B and all the pigs of group C. Lung lavage was performed under anaesthesia (30 mg sodium thiopental IV/kg). The animals were held in horizontal position, slightly inclined with the head upwards. A small plastic tube was passed into the trachea (about 20-25 cm) and 4x20 ml sterile saline solution was injected into the lung and immediately aspirated. The recovered saline solution was centrifuged. Both, serum and lung lavage fluids were tested for antibodies against ADV.

Challenge

Challenge of the pigs in groups B and C was performed by combined ON-IT route with $10^{7.5}$TCID$_{50}$ virulent ADV in 8 ml inoculum. In group B, 6 pigs were challenged at 1 month after the initial infection and 3 pigs at 2 months. Pigs were euthanized 0.5, 1, 2 or 3 days post challenge as indicated in Table 2. In group C, all the pigs were challenged 1 month after the last vaccination and they were euthanized 0.5,1,2 and 3 days later as indicated in Table 3. From all the euthanized pigs of groups A, B and C, tissue samples of the tonsils, nasal mucosae and diaphragmatic lung lobe were collected for virus titrations and immunofluorescence. Lavage of the other diaphragmatic lung lobe (with 100 ml saline solution) yielded the free cells from the air pathways, which were examined for virus quantity and by immunofluorescence.

Serology

The antibody titers in lung lavage fluids were determined in a sensitive seroneutralization test (Bitsch and Eskildsen, 1982). The fluids-virus mixtures were incubated for 24 hours at 37°C. Approximately 1 hour before bringing this mixture on a monolayer of a swine kidney (SK) cell line, 10 units of guinea pig complement were added. Titers are expressed as the reciprocal of the final dilution inhibiting cytopathic effect in 50% of the cultures.

The antibody titer of the sera was determined in a standard neutralization test.

Virus isolation and titrations

Virus titrations of the solid tissue specimens was performed on 20% tissue suspensions. Lung lavage fluids were centrifuged and the cell pellet, resuspended to obtain 10^7 cells/ml, was frozen and thawed twice to disrupt the cells and subsequently centrifuged. Virus titrations were performed in primary rabbit kidney monolayers according to standard procedures.

Immunofluorescence

A direct immunofluorescence method with a fluorescein isothiocyanate labeled anti-ADV serum was used on fresh tissue specimens and smears of free lung cells. Tissue specimens were frozen and subsequently cut with a cryostat. The sections, 8m thick, were fixed in acetone. Smears were dried and subsequently fixed in acetone. Sections and smears were stained with the conjugate according to standard procedures. The percentage positive alveolar macrophages was determined in the smears and the localization of the infected cells was examined in the tissue samples.

RESULTS

Virus isolations and titrations

The results of the virus titrations are presented in Tables 1,2,3. After ON inoculation of non-immune pigs (Table 1: group A_1), virus was recovered from all the inoculated pigs. In tonsils, titers of $10^{5.5}TCID_{50}/0.2$ g tissue and higher were consistently found. In the nasal mucosae, virus was recovered from 3 of the 4 pigs. In the lung tissue, virus was present but at low titers. Virus was isolated from the free lung cells in 2 of the 4 animals.

TABLE 1 Virus replication in tonsils and respiratory tract of susceptible feeder pigs after oronasal (A1) or intratracheal (A2) inoculation

Group	Killed (days pc)	Tonsils VT	Tonsils IF	Nasal mucosae VT	Nasal mucosae IF	Diaphragmatic lung lobe VT	Diaphragmatic lung lobe IF Br	IF br	IF Alv	Free cells of lung VT	Free cells of lung IF
A1	3	5.5	+	2.5	+	2.0	—	—	—	—	—
	4	5.7	+	4.7	—	5.5	—	—	+	3.3	+
	5	6.0	+	5.3	+	2.5	—	—	—	3.7	—
	7	6.0	+	—	—	1.0	—	—	+	—	—
A2	0.5	1.1	—	NT	NT	6.0	—	+	+	5.0	+
	0.5	1.0	—	NT	NT	6.5	—	+	+	5.0	+
	1	—	—	NT	NT	7.3	+	+	+	6.5	+
	2	5.5	+	NT	NT	>7.5	+	+	+	7.2	+
	2	4.5	+	NT	NT	7.3	+	+	+	5.7	+

VT:virus titers are expressed as $log_{10}TCID_{50}/0.2g$ tissue or $/10^7$ free lung cells
VT —means $<10^{0.6}TCID_{50}$; IF: immunofluorescence; IF +:positive; IF -:negative; pc: post challenge; NT: not tested; Br, br, Alv: Bronchi, bronchioli, alveoli, respectively.

After IT inoculation of non-immune pigs (Table 1: group A2), virus quantities in tonsils became high in later stages of the infection, starting at 2 days after inoculation. Lung tissue and the free cells contained virus titers which were very high as compared to those in the ON inoculated animals.

In the pigs, immune 1 and 2 months after infection (Table 2: groups B1 and 2) virus could not be detected in either tonsils or nasal mucosae. In the lungs and free cells, however, virus was still found but at much lower titers than in the non-immune animals. One month after infection (group B1), virus was isolated from from the lung in 3 of the 6 pigs euthanized at 0.5 and 1 days after challenge and from the free cells in 4 of the 6 pigs euthanized at 0.5, 1 and 2 days. Two months after infection (group B2) virus was again not recovered from nasal mucosae and tonsils, but was detected in the lung samples and free lung cells of all the pigs.

TABLE 2 Virus replication in tonsils and respiratory tract of feeder pigs upon combined oronasal-intratracheal challenge, 1 month (B1) and 2 months (B2) after previous infection

Group	Killed (days pc)	Virus titration (VT) and immunofluorescence (IF) in: Tonsils VT	Tonsils IF	Nasal mucosae VT	Nasal mucosae IF	Diaphragmatic lung lobe VT	Diaphragmatic lung lobe IF Br	IF br	IF Alv	Free cells of lung VT	Free cells of lung IF
B1	0.5	—	—	—	—	1.9	—	—	+	1.0	—
	0.5	—	—	—	—	2.0	—	—	+	1.0	+
	1	—	—	—	—	1.0	—	—	+	1.0	+
	2	—	—	—	—	—	—	—	+	—	—
	3	—	—	—	—	—	—	—	+	1.7	+
	3	—	—	—	—	—	—	—	—	—	—
B2	1	—	—	—	—	4.7	—	—	+	4.0	+
	2	—	—	—	—	1.9	—	+	+	4.0	+
	3	—	—	—	—	3.7	—	—	+	3.3	+

Legends: see Table 1;

From most of the pigs immune after vaccination (Table 3: group C1 and C2) challenge virus was recovered from tonsils, nasal mucosae and lungs. Virus replication was more widespread and occurred at higher titers in the pigs vaccinated with the live than in those vaccinated with the inactivated vaccine.

Immunofluorescence

The results are presented in Tables 1, 2 and 3. After ON inoculation of non-immune pigs (group A1), viral antigens were detected in all the tonsillar samples. Immunofluorescence was first observed in the crypt epithelial cells and the infection extended towards the cells of the lymphoid nodules beneath this epithelium. In the nasal mucosae, virus replication was demonstrated in some of the samples where the epithelial cells and subepithelial connective tissue were positive. Several sections (6 to 10) of tonsils and nasal mucosae had to be examined in some pigs to find some foci of cells containing viral antigen. Immunofluorescence in the lung parenchyma was not observed in all the pigs. In positive animals, it remained scarce and was limited to dispersed small foci of alveolar cells and interstitium. In one case, fluorescence was observed in alveolar macrophages of free cell smears.

TABLE 3 Virus replication in tonsils and respiratory tract of feeder pigs upon combined oronasal-intratracheal challenge, 1 month after last vaccination with inactivated (C1) or live (C2) vaccine.

Group	Killed (days pc)	Virus titration (VT) and immunofluorescence (IF) in										
		Tonsils		Nasal mucosae		Diaphragmatic lung lobe				Free cells of lung	
		VT	IF	VT	IF	VT	IF			VT	IF
							Br	br	Alv		
CI	0.5	—	+	—	—	3.3	—	—	+	NT	+
	1	0.8	+	0.6	—	5.5	+	+	+	NT	—
	2	—	+	1.7	+	4.7	—	+	+	NT	—
	3	2.7	+	4.0	+	—	—	+	+	NT	—
C2	0.5	—	—	1.7	—	5.0	—	+	+	3.5	+
	1	4.5	+	—	+	5.5	+	+	+	—	+
	2	5.2	+	5.0	+	6.2	—	+	+	3.5	+
	3	3.3	—	3.5	—	6.0	—	+	+	1.0	+
	3	4.7	+	4.5	+	3.5	—	+	+	—	—

Legends: see Table 1

In the lungs of IT inoculated non-immune pigs (group A2), virus replication at 0.5, 1 and 2 days involved less than 10%, between 10%-50% and more than 50% of the lung tissue, respectively. At 0.5 days post challenge, fluorescence was observed in epithelial cells of terminal bronchioli, in alveolar cells, interstitial cells and alveolar macrophages. At 1 and 2 days, bronchi and bronchioli were also infected with fluorescence present in the epithelial cells and in the underlying connective tissue.

In pigs immune after infection (groups B1 and B2), viral antigens were not detected in tonsils or nasal mucosae. Virus replication in lung tissue was limited to alveolar cells, interstitial cells and alveolar macrophages and less than 10% of the lung parenchyma was infected in each of the pigs. Epithelial cells of bronchioli were seldom positive.

In pigs immune after vaccination with an inactivated vaccine (group C1), replication of the challenge virus was seen in tonsillar crypt epithelial cells of all the pigs and in lymphoid tissue of 1 animal. In nasal mucosae, viral antigens were observed in a few clusters of epithelial cells in 2 of the 4 pigs. In the lungs, fluorescence was mainly seen in alveolar cells and interstitium, but viral antigens were also observed in the epithelial cells of bronchi in 1 pig and in the epithelial cells of bronchioli in 2 pigs.

In the pigs immune after vaccination with an attenuated vaccine (group C2), replication of challenge virus was seen in tonsillar crypts of 3 of the 5 pigs. In nasal mucosae, viral antigens were observed in epithelial cells of 3 pigs, but also in subepithelial connective tissue of 1 pig.

Virus replication in the lung involved maximum 10% at 0.5 day and between 10% and 50% at 1, 2 and 3 days post challenge. In the lung tissue, alveolar cells, interstitial cells and alveolar macrophages were positive as well as epithelial cells of bronchioli; epithelial cells of bronchi were seldom positive. Subepithelial connective tissue also was fluorescing in some bronchioli in the pig euthanized at 2 days post challenge.

In smears of lung lavage, alveolar macrophages were fluorescing in some pigs in each of the groups as indicated in Tables 1,2 and 3. The number of positive cells did not exceed 1%, except in 2 pigs, and a difference between non-immune and immune pigs was not evident.

Serology

Before infection or vaccination, all the pigs were free of antibodies against ADV in their serum. Before inoculation lung lavage fluid of the pigs tested were negative.

Four weeks after infection, antibody titers were seen in the serum of all the pigs. Titers varied from 48 to 192 (geometric mean titer - GMT of 84.4). All the lung lavage samples of these pigs contained antibodies with titers varying from 2 to 6 (GMT: 3.2). Serum titers in pigs vaccinated with the inactivated vaccine varied between 12 and 32 (GMT: 19.6) and 3 lung lavage samples were negative (<2), whereas 1 sample had a titer of 2.

After vaccination with the attenuated vaccine, serum titers were <2 in 2 pigs and varied from 4 to 24 (GMT: 6.0) in the other 3 pigs, but in none of the lung lavage samples antibodies were detected.

DISCUSSION

In the present study, an insight into the sites and cell types of virus replication with ADV in the respiratory tract was sought. First, susceptible pigs were inoculated oronasally, but the infection pattern obtained in the lungs of these pigs was erratic and insufficiently reproducible to be used for comparison in studying the sequence of events which occurs in immune animals. The intratracheal inoculation with a high virus dose was, therefore, tested out. This route of inoculation resulted in susceptible pigs in a consistently high degree of infection in the lungs. Even though the number of pigs used in the present study was too low to make firm conclusions, it was clear that the infection started in cells of the alveoli and terminal bronchioli and that free bronchio-alveolar cells supported virus replication at high titers. The present studies provided evidence that these free cells and particularly virus containing alveolar macrophages, present in the lumen of the air pathways, play an important role in the dissemination of ADV in the respiratory tract.

The present studies also confirmed previous findings that the amount of virus which enters the respiratory tract at once is important to determine the evolution of the infection in the lungs. The intratracheal inoculation resulted in a widespread infection throughout the lungs, whereas the infection remained limited to few foci after oronasal inoculation. Massive infection of bronchio-alveolar macrophages likely decreases the important non-specific defence mechanisms in the air pathways.

Because the present work was designed to study the sequence of events of the infection in immune pigs and to compare it with that in susceptible pigs, a combined oronasal-intratracheal challenge route was selected. This way, virus was introduced at the same time at the different replication sites in the respiratory tract and a reproducible infection pattern was obtained.

Even though it has repeatedly been shown that virus replication upon challenge still can occur in the respiratory tract of ADV-vaccinated pigs, it was remarkable that replication also took place in solidly immune pigs, already 1 month after previous infection with virulent virus.

That virus replication was totally prevented in nasal mucosa and tonsils of pigs immune after previous infection points to a good mucosal immunity at these sites. However, this mucosal protection was absent or insufficient in vaccinated animals, even 1 month after intranasal vaccination. Since natural infection with ADV in pigs mainly occurs by aerogenic route, the lack of protection in vaccinated pigs at these superficial sites of entry may be problematic in attempts to eradicate ADV by vaccination, even if such vaccination would be carried out strictly. Of course, the challenge dose used in the present studies was higher than the dose of infection under natural conditions, but the results of the fluorescence showed that invasion of both nasal mucosa and tonsils in vaccinated pigs occurs rather easily.

The findings in the lungs of the immune pigs were quite interesting. Both in the 1 and 2 months infection-immune animals, virus replication occurred in the lungs. The only cell types involved in the early infection stages were intraluminal free cells and cells in the alveoli. Even though it is difficult to prove, evidence was present that alveolar macrophages became primarily infected. These cells may well have been responsible for carrying the virus to the alveolar cells through cell to cell contact. Apparently, alveolar macrophages are susceptible to ADV independently of the immune status of the animal. The amount of virus entering the deeper air pathways possibly together with the presence or absence of antibodies may well be important to determine whether alveolar macrophages become infected or not in immune animals.

Apparently, once the infection has started, it is of shorter duration. Unpublished observations in our laboratory have shown that, shortly after the infection in the lungs has began, numerous neutrophils are invading the air pathways. It can be supposed that these cells can terminate the infection rather quickly through antibody dependent cellular cytotoxicity, since neutrophils are known to be good effector cells in this process (Ashworth *et al.,* 1979). Whatever immunity mechanisms take place, it was clear that their efficiency to limit the infection was much less in the lungs of vaccinated pigs than in those of infection-immune animals. Again, this finding indicates that eradication of ADV through vaccination may be a difficult task.

Antibodies in the air pathways of animals immune to ADV are probably important not only to prevent infection but also to limit it. Such antibodies, detected with the highly sensitive seroneutralisation test, were consistently present in lavage fluids of infection-immune animals. We believe that their presence is directly correlated with a short lasting infection in the lungs of immune pigs. With other virus infections of the respiratory tract, such as with swine influenza virus, infection can totally be prevented in animals immune after vaccination with an inactivated vaccine even if a heavy intratracheal challenge is administered (Haesebrouck and Pensaert, 1986). A vaccination schedule which induces high antibody titers in the air pathways either by local antibody formation or by transudation from the serum, may be necessary to meet success in ADV eradication attempts. It is doubtful that sufficiently high antibody titers can be obtained in the air pathways with live ADV vaccines even if intranasally administered. Frequent injections with immunologically potent inactivated vaccines, inducing high serum titers, may well be optimal to limit infection in the lung tissue.

A local immunity at the upper primary replication sites (nasal mucosa, tonsils) combined with the presence of antibodies in the deeper air pathways may well be essential to eradicate ADV by vaccination programmes. Whether this combination can be obtained in a practical way is another question!

ACKNOWLEDGEMENTS

These studies were carried out with the financial support of the Institute for the Encouragement of Research in Industry and Agriculture (IWONL), Brussels, Belgium.

The technical assistance of Mrs. C. Van Maercke and Mr. A. Van der Beken was gratefully appreciated.

REFERENCES

Andries, K., Pensaert, M.B. and Vandeputte, J. 1978. Effect of experimental infection with Pseudorabies (Aujeszky's disease) virus on pigs with maternal immunity from vaccinated sows. Am.J.Vet.Res., **39**, 1282-1285.

Ashworth, L.A.E., Lloyd, G. and Baskerville, A. 1979. Antibody-dependent cell mediated cytotoxicity (ADCC) in Aujeszky's disease. Arch.Virol., **59**, 307-318.

Baskerville, A. 1973. Ultrastructural changes in the lungs of pigs infected with Aujeszky's disease virus. Res.Vet.Sci., **14**, 229-233.

Bitsch, V. and Eskildsen, M. 1982. Complement dependent neutralization of Aujeszky's disease virus by antibody. Curr.Top.Vet.Med.Anim.Sci., **17**, 41-49. Proc. CEC Seminar "Aujeszky's disease", Tübingen 1981 (Ed. G. Wittman and S.A. Hall).

De Leeuw, P.W. and Van Oirschot, J.T. 1985. Vaccines against Aujeszky's disease: evaluation of their efficacy under standardized laboratory. Vet. Quart., **7**, 191-197.

Donaldson, A.I., Wardley, R.C., Martin, S. and Harkness, J.W. 1984. Influence of vaccination on Aujeszky's disease virus and disease transmission. Vet.Rec., **115**, 121-124.

Haesebrouck, F. and Pensaert, M.B. 1986. Effect of intratracheal challenge of fattening pigs previously immunized with an inactivated influenza H_1N_1 vaccine. Vet. Microbiol., **11**, 239-249.

Maes, L., Haesebrouck, F. and Pensaert, M.B. 1984. Experimental reproduction of clinical disease by intratracheal inoculation of fattening pigs with swine influenza isolates. Proc. 8th Congr. Int.Pig.Vet.Soc. Ghent, 60.

McFerran, J.B., Dow, C. and McCracken, R.M. 1979. Experimental studies with three vaccines against Aujeszky's disease. Comp.Immun.Microbiol.Infect.Dis., **2**, 327-334.

Pensaert, M.B. and Maes, L. 1984. Parenteral and intranasal vaccination of fattening pigs against Aujeszky's disease virus (Pseudorabies). Zbl.Vet.Med.B, **33,** 682-689.

Wittmann, G., Jakubik, J. and Ahl, R. 1980. Multiplication and distribution of Aujeszky's disease virus in vaccinated and non-vaccinated pigs after intranasal infection. Arch.Virol., **66,** 227-240.

Wittmann, G., Ohlinger, V. and Höhn, U. 1982. Vermehrung von Aujeszkyvirus (AV) in vakzinierten Schweinen nach experimenteller Infektion mit hohen und niederer Virusmengen. Zbl.Vet.Med. B, **29,** 24-30.

Van Oirschot, J.T. and Gielkens, A.L.J. 1987. Vaccines against Aujeszky's disease: comparison of efficacy, DNA fingerprints and antibody response to glycoprotein I. Vet.Quart.,**9,** S37-S49.

THE CONTROL AND ERADICATION OF AUJESZKY'S DISEASE IN DENMARK: EPIDEMIOLOGICAL ASPECTS

J.B. Andersen, V. Bitsch**, L.S. Christensen***, R. Hoff-Jørgensen****, B. Kirkegaard Petersen******

*Danish Veterinary Service, Frederiksgade 21, DK-1265 Copenhagen K, Denmark
**Danish Dairy Board, Frederiks Allé 22, DK-8000 Århus C, Denmark
***State Veterinary Institute for Virus Research, Lindholm, DK-4771 Kalvehave, Denmark
****National Veterinary Laboratory, Bülowsvej 27, Postboks 373, DK-1503 Copenhagen V, Denmark
*****Danish Bacon and Meat Council, Axelborg, Axeltorv 3, DK-1609 Copenhagen V, Denmark

ABSTRACT

The appearance of more pathogenic strains of Aujeszky's disease (AD) virus (ADV) during the late seventies and these strains' liability for airborne transmission is reviewed and a description of the control- and eradication program introduced in 1980 is given. It is concluded that the chosen infection control strategy has been efficient and that AD in reality was eradicated in the autumn 1986. However, during the winter and spring of 1986-1987 and 1987-1988 a series of outbreaks have taken place in the southern part of Jutland and in Funen. All infected herds have been removed and an area around the outbreaks was screened in 1987 and will again be screened in 1988. The epidemiological examinations including restriction-fragment-pattern (RFP) analysis of the isolates strongly indicate that these outbreaks were caused by a reintroduction of the infection and not by a reactivation. These experiences also give strong evidence that ADV under certain conditions can be transmitted airborne over much longer distances than realized so far. The findings emphasize the importance and the need for an international cooperation on the control of AD.

INTRODUCTION

Aujeszky's Disease (AD) has been known to exist in Denmark since 1931, when the disease occurred in cattle, and it has been recognized as a disease entity in pigs since 1964. Until the late seventies the disease did not cause severe losses. In cattle, only sporadic cases in single animals were seen. In pigs, only piglets showed clinical disease and mortality, with a degree of natural immunity being built up in the rest of the herd.

J. T. van Oirschot (ed.), Vaccination and Control of Aujeszky's Disease, 175–183.

However, from 1978 onwards an increasing number of severe outbreaks of AD was recorded. In infected pig herds abortions of infected fetuses became a normal clinical manifestation in addition to an increased mortality rate in young pigs and even in adult animals.

Fattening pigs often showed respiratory symptoms, and where cattle were kept close to infected pigs severe outbreaks with more infected animals were now recorded. In such cases the animals showed anterior pruritus (paraesthesia) and virus could often be isolated from the respiratory tract, indicating a respiratory infection.

During the same period the Danish pig industry has undergone an intensive development, with decrease in the number of small herds and increase in the size of production herds as well as breeding herds.

PATHOGENICITY OF VIRUS STRAINS

From a study on differences between strains of AD virus (ADV) it was found that strains isolated from severe outbreaks in swine and cattle i.e. outbreaks with abortions and high mortality in pig herds and anterior pruritus in more animals in cattle herds, would regularly cause syncytia-forming degeneration of cell cultures, in contract to strains isolated from less severe outbreaks, which would cause round-cell-degeneration (Bitsch, 1980).

About 60% of the isolates from outbreaks in pig herds in 1982 was found to be syncytia-forming, as against about 50% in 1980 and 1981 and about 20% in 1978 and 1979. These findings reflected the above mentioned change in the disease situation and supported the assumption of the appearance of more virulent virus strains.

TRANSMISSION OF VIRUS

Until 1978 the main conclusion was that herds got infected because of direct contact with pigs shedding virus during the acute infection phase or during a later period after reactivation of the infection. After the appearance of highly pathogenic strains of the virus, however, this general point of view could no longer be strictly maintained, as outbreaks caused by syncytia-forming strains often occurred in herds, where no immediate contact with animals from infected herds was imaginable. Two possible explanations of the introduction of the infection in such cases were conceivable: either transmission by rodents or airborne herd-to-herd spread of the virus.

The question was whether infection with especially syncytia-forming virus strains could be established in a mouse or at population. In experiments (Bitsch, unpublished observation) with young mice infected nasally, the inoculated animals regularly died, while in-contact mice survived and were susceptible to challenge infection. Similar results were obtained with young rats. When relatively low virus doses were used, some rats survived, but they did not resist subsequent challenge infection. The conclusions were the same for both syncytia-forming and non-syncytia-forming strains: mice and rats were susceptible and would die, if they were infected, but the infection was not easily established. These findings were consistent with those obtained by others (Kirkpatrick *et al.*, 1980), and did not seem to support the idea of a herd-to-herd spread of the infection by rodents.

The first observations indicating airborne transmission were made in cases, where cattle standing in an airflow from infected pigs, e.g. a pig barn with open doors or windows into the cow barn, were infected by the inhalation route, and where the outbreaks in cattle stopped as soon as the airflow from the pigs was interrupted (Bitsch and Andersen, 1982). This illustrates the fact that ventilators in a pig house with an acutely infected herd will blow considerable amounts of virus out into the open air. It was difficult based on the above observation to estimate the risk of an airborne herd-to-herd transmission, but logically it would depend on the efficiency of the ventilation system, the size of both the infected and the uninfected herd, weather conditions, and the characteristics of the virus strain.

However, during the control and eradication campaign, we have, under specific weather conditions (wind direction, high humidity, low temperature), seen a great many cases where airborne transmission over up to 2-3 kilometers seems to be the only possible explanation for the spread of the disease. These observations are consistent with findings later reported from Great Britain (Gloster *et al.*, 1984). It is noteworthy that the infection in most of the above cases seems to have spread from herds with fattening pigs, as the clinical symptoms in acutely infected fattening pigs are often combined with respiratory distress and coughing, which must increase the amount of airborne virus.

THE CONTROL AND ERADICATION PROGRAM

Owing to the changed disease situation we had to decide on a new strategy for the control of AD in Denmark. Knowing the costs of a full vaccination program and knowing that the export potential as well as the efficiency of production would be threatened by the continued existence of AD, the decision was taken to completely eliminate the infectious agent from the Danish national herd. This was considered feasible because the elite breeding herds had already been cleared for AD-infection, the boar stations (artificial insemination) were free of AD and the geographical division of Denmark into well-separated regions facilitated the effectuation of movements controls and regional control programs. In addition, the available serological test-method was considered sensitive and specific enough to be used with confidence in an eradication program. In the beginning of the program a modified virus-serum neutralization test (Bitsch and Eskildsen, 1976) was used. This test was from 1983 with the increasing number of samples to be examined replaced by a blocking ELISA test (Sørensen and Lei, 1986).

The AD control and eradication program was introduced in April 1980, when AD was made notifiable, and has followed the conventional principles for infection control programs carried out under Danish conditions, starting from a voluntary accreditation scheme encouraging the trading of AD-free animals only, through increasing regional restrictions, cleaning-up of low-prevalence areas, and finally extending the program to comprise compulsory testing of all herds and the introduction of heavy restrictions on all infected premises in the country. In pursuance of the latest AD Order (December 15, 1987) pigs removed from an infected herd must go directly to a slaughterhouse or to an incinerating plant, and the transport has to be carried out without contact to pigs from AD-free herds. Furthermore, no pigs are permitted entry into an infected herd, and the Danish Veterinary Service is entitled to prescribe rules for the handling of liquid manure, bedding material and fodder from such a herd. Vaccination against AD has never been practiced and has from 1983 been prohibited.

The eradication has been carried out in close cooperation with the industry. From the beginning of the program the Danish Bacon and Meat Council (DBMC) has paid the laboratory costs of the serological examinations for AD. From January 1983 DBMC has subsidized a "slaughtering out" of infected herds after acute outbreak and from June 1983 also a "test and slaughter" clearing of latently infected herds. Funds were generated for this by the imposition of a levy administered by DBMC on all pigs slaughtered. Together with the latest tightening up of the national rules (April 1985) DBMC has imposed a charge on pigs delivered for slaughter from herds not considered free of AD.

The current surveillance of AD is based on the following systems:

1. AD is notifiable. Acutely infected herds being removed (subsidized by DBMC), and a screening of an approximately 10 km area around the outbreak being carried out.

2. Testing of all breeding boars and boars over 100 kg (body weight) at slaughter or at export.
3. Follow-up testing of herds every 2 years.
a. 15% of the adult animals in breeding and mixed breeding-feeder herds.
b. 5% of the animals in pure feeder units.
4. Monthly testing of travelling boars.

RESULTS

The monitoring system using breeding boars as sentinel animals among the entire pig population was first introduced in February 1981 for the island of Bornholm (AD-free), but has since October 1983 covered the whole country. In 1984, 29,323 boars have been sampled and the trace-back of positive boars has lead to the registration of 142 herds not previously known to be infected. The figures for 1985, 1986 and 1987 are 29,845, 33,772 and 32,102 sampled boars and 24, 5 and 0 disclosed herds, respectively.

The change through the phases of the program of the overall prevalence based on the official herd status has previously been described in details (Andersen, 1984, 1986). The similar pictures obtained from the official boar monitoring data and the herd testing data and showing a nearly linear decline to zero have also been demonstrated. At the end of 1986 only 32 herds out of a total number of 47,814 herds were registered as infected with AD. These herds were generally small herds with 1 or 2 seroreacting animals and in most cases the seroreactors were already slaughtered.

The travelling boar tradition in Denmark goes way back and in 1980, after which year new enterprises with travelling boars could no longer be established, 163 such enterprises were recorded. Along with the restrictions on travelling boars implemented as part of the AD-eradication program, the number of such enterprises has dropped markedly and today only 25 are left.

TABLE 1 Virologically confirmed outbreaks of Aujeszky's Disease, 1978 - May 1988

	1978	**79**	**80**	**81**	**82**	**83**	**84**	**85**	**86**	**87**	**88** (first 5 months)
Swine	62	67	83	65	89	105	46	38	2	10	43
Cattle	8	9	8	19	13	13	6	5	—	—	2
Dogs	1	2	5	4	6	6	1	3	—	—	—
Cats	—	—	1	3	1	6	1	2	—	—	—
Red Foxes	5	5	4	5	9	4	2	1	—	—	—

The number of outbreaks confirmed by virus isolation since 1978 are shown in Table 1, and the localization of the outbreaks during the period January 1985 - May 1988 is shown in Fig. 1.

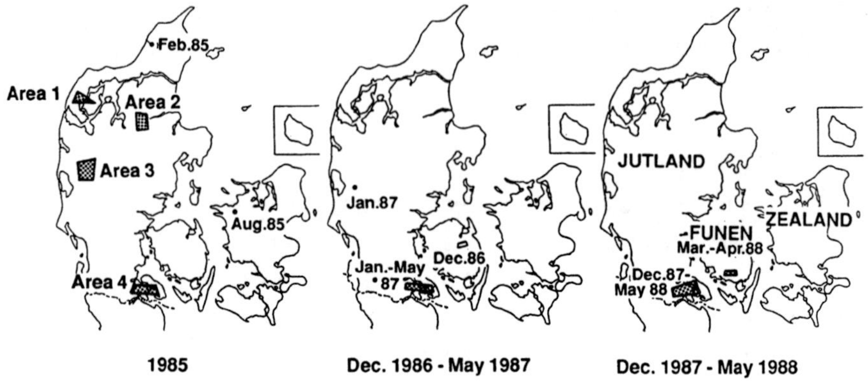

Fig. 1 Localization of virologically confirmed AD-outbreaks 1985-1988

In the period November 1985 - December 1986 no outbreaks were recorded. However, in December 1986 2 outbreaks occurred in Funen and later in January 1987 1 single outbreak in Mid-Jutland and in January - May 1987 7 outbreaks in South-Jutland were reported. After a silent period in the summer and autumn 1987, 47 outbreaks have been reported during December 1987 and the first 5 months of 1988.

The outbreaks have since 1984 been characterized by being, geographically and in time, limited epizooties, as illustrated in Fig. 1. The few single outbreaks (North-Jutland February 1985, Zealand August 1985 and Mid-Jutland January 1987) did all occur in small herds and these outbreaks are, according to the epidemiological investigations, considered as results of reactivation of infection with relatively low-virulent strains. The outbreaks in 1985 occurred in 4 areas in Jutland, but since 1986 the outbreaks have been limited to Funen and to the south-eastern part of Jutland. The epidemiological investigations of the first outbreaks in 1986-1987 and 1987-1988 revealed no evidence of any contact, which could explain the emergence of the disease.

After the outbreaks in 1985 and in 1986-1987 an area of approximately 10 kilometers around the outbreaks was screened. A few reactors were found. These reactors were slaughtered and the herds were retested at least 3 weeks after removal of the reactors. A screening of the southern part of Funen and the south-eastern part of Jutland is planned to be carried out later in 1988.

IDENTIFICATION OF VIRUS

ADV strains can to a certain extent be differentiated through restriction fragment pattern (RFP) analysis of their genomes (DNA-fingerprinting), and this method is considered a very valuable tool for the epidemiological investigations. Examinations carried out at the State Veterinary Institute for Virus Research, Lindholm (Christensen *et al.*, 1987; Christensen and Sørensen, 1988) have shown that virus isolates from Danish AD-outbreaks up to 1985 represented a genome type, which is characteristic for Danish strains only. However, 7 out of 42 virus strains isolated from Danish outbreaks in 1985 belonged to a genome type (Group II), which is widespread in Central-Europe (Herrmann *et al.*, 1984), but was never previously found in Danish isolates. These outbreaks occurred in January-February 1985 in the south-eastern part of Jutland (Area 4 in Fig. 1) close to the Danish-German border.

The virus isolates from the outbreaks in 1986-1987 and the virus isolates examined so far from the outbreaks in 1987-1988 all belong to the same Central-European genome type (Group II). According to a further development of the classification system, Group II can now be divided into subgroups, and it is found (Christensen *et al.*, 1988) that the isolates from the winter 1986-1987 and the Group II isolates from January-February 1985 all belong to Subgroup IIa, whereas the first 8 isolates from the winter 1987-1988 belong to Subgroup IIp, which has never previously been found in Danish isolates.

Eight isolates collected during the period May-October 1987 from AD-outbreaks in the region Schleswig-Flensburg, the Federal Republic of Germany and kindly provided by Direktor Dr. Th. Zimmermann, Veterinäruntersuchungsamt des Landes Schleswig-Holstein, Neumünster have been found to belong to Subgroup IIa and IIp, with 6 and 2 isolates, respectively.

DISCUSSION

Considering a) that Denmark on December 1, 1986 had been without outbreaks of AD for more than 1 year, b) that all Danish pig herds had been tested serologically, c) that only a few herds were not registered as officially AD-free and finally considering d) that the surveillance programs had revealed no new infected herds during 1986, it can be concluded that the implemented infection control strategy has been efficient and that AD in reality was eradicated from the Danish territory in the autumn 1986.

Remembering that ADV is a herpesvirus, it was likely that not all infected animals had been discovered, and that a reactivation of the infection in a latently infected animal, not discovered by the surveillance system, had to be calculated on as a risk. However, the above mentioned AD-free position combined with the screening around all outbreaks in 1985 and in 1986-1987 together with the localization of the outbreaks indicate that the first outbreaks in the winter 1986-1987 and again in the winter 1987-1988 were caused by new introduction of the infection and not by a reactivation of a national source of infection. This conclusion is strongly supported by the results of the RFP-analyses.

As the epidemiological investigations revealed no evidence of any contact, which could explain the emergence of the infection, it can also be concluded that the disease most likely has been transmitted airborne from outbreaks south of the border. This conclusion is supported by the experiences made during the introduction and spread in 1984-1986 of a TGE-like airborne porcine coronavirus (Andersen *et al.*, 1986) which followed an equal pattern.

Vannier and Le Foll (1987) have, when comparing the actions taken against AD in Europe, emphasized the importance of a cooperation between the European countries particularly for the trade in breeding animals with harmonized control measures and for the protection of countries considered as free of AD. The recent Danish experiences have also demonstrated the importance and the urgent need for such cooperation.

REFERENCES

Andersen, J.B. 1984. Measures for the control of Aujeszky's disease in Denmark. In: 11th Conference of the O.I.E. Regional Commission for Europe, Vienna, pp.375-380.

Andersen, J.B. 1986. Use of abattoirs as a source of epidemiological data. In: 12th Conference of the O.I.E. Regional Commission for Europe, Berlin-East, pp.199-206.

Andersen, J.B., Eskildsen, M. and Kirkegaard Petersen, B. 1986. AEndring i de lovmæssige bestemmelser for TGE-virus infektioner. Dansk Vet. Tidsskr., **69**, 471-473.

Bitsch, V. 1980. Correlation between the pathogenicity of field strains of Aujeszky's disease virus and their ability to cause cell fusion - syncytia-formation - in cell cultures. Acta Vet. Scand., **21**, 708-710.

Bitsch, V. and Andersen, J.B. 1982. On the epidemiology of Aujeszky's disease in Denmark and the possibilities of its control. Ref.: Curr. Top. Vet. Anim. Sci., **17**, 227-236. In: CEC Seminar on "Aujeszky's disease" (Eds. G. Wittmann and S.A. Hall). (Martinus Nijhoff, The Hague).

Bitsch, V. and Eskildsen, M. 1976. A comparative examination of swine sera for antibody to Aujeszky virus with the conventional and a modified virus-serum neutralization test and a modified direct complement fixation test. Acta Vet. Scand., **17**, 142-152.

Christensen, L.S., Sørensen, K.J. and Lei, J.C. 1987. Restriction fragment pattern (RFP) analysis of genomes from Danish isolates of suid herpesvirus 1 (Aujeszky's disease virus). Arch. Virol., **97**, 215-224.

Christensen, L.S. and Sørensen, K.J. 1988. Introduction of foreign strains of suid herpesvirus pattern (RFP) analysis. Arch. Virol., **100**, 109-113.

Christensen, L.S., Sørensen, K.J., Lei, J.C., Andersen, J.B. and Henriksen, C.A. 1988. Aujeszky's sygdom: Den epizootiologiske situation belyst ved restriktionsfragmentmönsterannalyser. Dansk Vet. Tidsskr. (in press).

Gloster, J., Donaldson, A.J. and Hough, M.N. 1984. Analysis of a series of outbreaks of Aujeszky's disease in York in 1981-1982: The possibility of airborne disease spread. Vet. Rec., **114**, 234-239.

Herrmann, S.C., Heppner, B. and Ludwig, H. 1984. Pseudorabies virus from clinical outbreaks and latent infections grouped into four major genome types. Ref.: Curr. Top. Vet. Anim. Sci., **27**, 387-401. In: CEC Seminar on "Latent herpesvirus Infections in Veterinary Medicine" (Eds. G. Wittmann, R.M. Gaskell and H.J. Rziha). (Martinus Nijhoff, The Hague).

Kirkpatrick, C.M., Kanitz, C.L. and McCrocklin, S.M. 1980. Possible role of wild mammals in transmission of pseudorabies to swine. J. Wildlife Dis., **16**, 601-614.

Sørensen, K.J. and Lei, J.C. 1986. Aujeszky's Disease: Blocking ELISA for the detection of serum antibodies. J. Virol. Method., **13**, 171-181.

Vannier, P and Le Foll, P. 1987. Comparing actions against Aujeszky's disease in Europe. Pig International, **17**, 18-24.

EPIDEMIOLOGICAL ASPECTS OF AUJESZKY'S DISEASE CONTROL IN GREAT BRITAIN

K.C. Taylor

Ministry of Agriculture, Fisheries and Food, Hook Rise South
Tolworth, Surbiton, Surrey, KT6 7NF, England

ABSTRACT

Aujeszky's disease was first recorded in Great Britain in 1953. Outbreaks of severe clinical disease were seen in pigs from 1971. The number of affected herds was small, not exceeding 16 in any year until the disease was made notifiable in 1979. An industry-financed programme to control and eradicate Aujeszky's disease started in March 1983 and is still continuing. The number of confirmed outbreaks has been reduced from 443 in 1983 to 6 in 1987. Most outbreaks are confirmed on serological evidence only, and clinical disease is now rarely seen. Despite 3 linked clinical outbreaks confirmed early in 1988 serological surveillance results encourage the belief that the goal of eradication may be near.

The epidemiological features of Aujeszky's disease in Great Britain, observed before and during the eradication campaign, are described and illustrated by specific examples. The movement of subclinically infected pigs, particularly from the minority of breeding units on which management standards are poor, has been the most frequent method by which infection has spread. Breeding movements, particularly those involving the use of communal boars, have also been important. The significance of airborne spread has generally been difficult to determine, although a series of outbreaks in which airborne virus caused infection up to 9 km from the source has been described. There has been little evidence to suggest the reactivation of latent infection. Serological studies of subclinically infected herds, including those which have not spread infection when selling pigs, suggest the continued spread of infection amongst adult sows and boars.

HISTORY OF AUJESZKY'S DISEASE IN BRITAIN

Aujeszky's disease (AD) was first diagnosed in Great Britain amongst pigs in South-West England in 1953. Subsequent outbreaks were sporadic and mainly affected cattle and sheep, with pigs showing little evidence of clinical disease until the late 1960s, from which time the number and severity of recorded outbreaks increased slowly.

Until AD was made notifiable in August 1979 the number of newly infected herds identified in any year had never exceeded 16. Even if allowance is made for unreported cases having occurred it is clear that the number of affected herds was

J. T. van Oirschot (ed.), Vaccination and Control of Aujeszky's Disease, 185–196.

small, and certainly not comparable with the numbers occurring in some continental European countries at that time. When the disease was made notifiable the number of confirmed outbreaks confirmed in the year increased to 34 (Fig. 1).

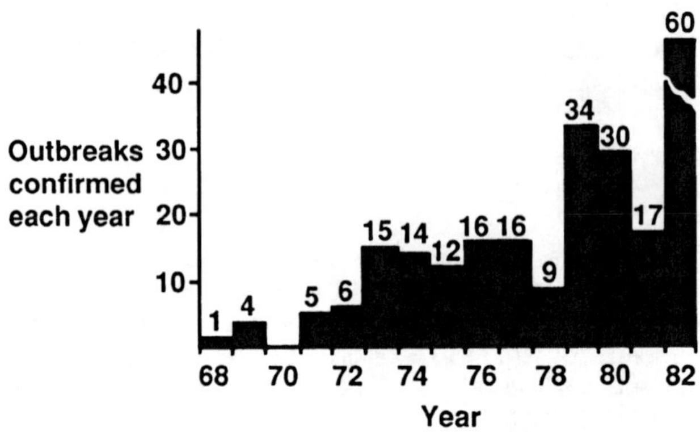

Fig. 1 Newly infected AD premises 1968-1982

Although Aujeszky's disease (AD) in pigs was made notifiable in 1979 no other official action was taken at that time. A stamping-out policy was considered - and rejected - in 1980, but the number of outbreaks continued to increase, reaching a peak of 60 in 1982. A survey of 12500 sera collected from pigs at slaughter that year confirmed the impression that infection was continuing to spread amongst British pig herds, and the situation was again reviewed. Assuming continued spread at the same rate it was estimated that if no action was taken 1000 herds would be infected by 1985, and up to 3000 by 1990. Various strategies for dealing with the disease were again considered and it was concluded that stamping out was now the strategy of choice, compensation being paid for all pigs slaughtered and healthy pigs salvaged for human consumption. A poll of pig keepers in November 1982 gave overwhelming support for a control and eradication programme financed by the industry by means of a statutory levy of 30p payable for every pig slaughtered for human consumption.

New legislation was necessary to provide the State Veterinary Service with the powers required to implement the programme, in particular:

a. Requiring the notification of suspended disease, either on clinical grounds or as a result of laboratory tests.

b. Authorizing the imposition of restrictions on premises on which there were suspected pigs.

c. Requiring the State Veterinary Service to investigate all reports of suspected disease, and the Chief Veterinary Officer to confirm the existence of disease.
d. Allowing the valuation and slaughter of pigs with payment of compensation.
e. Authorizing the tracing and investigation of contact pigs in other herds.
f. Requiring cleansing and disinfection of infected premises.
g. Authorizing the State Veterinary Service to maintain restrictions on premises until satisfied that infection no longer existed.

These powers were contained in the Aujeszky's Disease Order 1983 and the Aujeszky's Disease (Compensation for Swine) Order 1983, both of which came into operation on 10th March 1983. The Control and Eradication Programme started on 14th March 1983.

THE AUJESZKY'S DISEASE CONTROL AND ERADICATION PROGRAMME

The first stage of the programme involved resampling the 220 herds already known to have been infected, tracing movements to and from infected herds and blood sampling every herd within 2 km of a confirmed outbreak. AD was re-confirmed in 118 of the previously known infected herds: the others had either been depopulated, or infection had been eliminated from the herd. AD was also confirmed in 312 other herds as a result of movement tracing and area patrols so that, on completion of this stage on 30th September 1983, 430 infected herds had been dealt with and 341,000 pigs slaughtered. In the course of dealing with these outbreaks more than 3,300 investigations were undertaken and 94,000 blood samples collected for serological testing. Of the 312 previously unknown infected herds 22 had been notified as suspected disease, 155 were identified by tracing and 135 by 2 km patrols (Animal Health 1983: Report of the Chief Veterinary Officer).

Having completed stage I it had to be assumed that in spite of all the tracing and patrol sampling carried out undiscovered foci of infection would still exist. The aim of the second stage - which is still continuing - is to seek out the remaining infected herds, and so progress to the eventual eradication of AD. The disease is notifiable and suspected outbreaks of clinical disease continue to be investigated. Additionally it was decided to organise serum surveys to seek evidence of sero-conversion.

A variety of surveys have been undertaken, but the main emphasis has been on cull sows sampled at slaughterhouses. About 400,000 sows are culled each year and Table 1 shows the number of samples examined and the percentage found to be positive. A study of serological results in herds in which disease had been confirmed indicated boars to be as effective for monitoring as sows, and the routine sow survey was discontinued on 31 December 1987. Regular surveillance is now concentrated on cull boars, the intention being to sample every breeding boar at slaughter. Statistical returns indicate that 15,000 of the 40,000 breeding boars in the country are culled each year: in the 5 months to 31st May 1988, 8789 had been sampled, all with negative results. Sow surveys are still undertaken intermittently, the intention being to sample every sow slaughtered during a specified 4 week period. One such intensive exercise has been undertaken in 1988: the results are included in Table 1.

TABLE 1 Cull sow serum survey 1984-1988

Year	Samples	Positive incidents	%positive
1984	38,510	36	0.093
1985	65,461	58	0.089
1986	69,048	13	0.019
1987	53,655	5	0.009
1988 (intensive period)	20,942	1	0.005
Totals	247,616	113	

Positive samples identified at slaughterhouses are traced and pigs on the premises of origin are blood sampled. Serological evidence of infection is not invariably found, but where disease is confirmed pigs on the premises are slaughtered and an epidemiological investigation undertaken: movements on and off are traced to identify origin and spread of infection, and a 2 km patrol sampling undertaken. Most disease outbreaks are confirmed on serological evidence only: clinical disease is rarely seen. Table 2 shows the number of outbreaks confirmed each year and indicates the reasons for initially visiting those herds. The importance of serum surveys has been even greater than the figures indicate, particularly in recent years, since some outbreaks identified by tracing would not have been visited if slaughterhouse surveillance had not identified the index case.

The recent reappearance of acute clinical disease in 3 herds in Cheshire has been an unexpected setback, and a salutory reminder about the continuing risk posed by undiscovered infected herds. Despite this setback surveillance results remain encouraging, and the goal of eradication may be near. The net cost to the industry has been about £26 million: more than expected, but excellent value if eradication is achieved.

TABLE 2 Number of outbreaks of AD confirmed each year, and reason for initial visit to each.

Reason for visit	1983	1984	1985	1986	1987	1988*
Reported disease	22	6	1	0	0	2
2 km patrol	139	7	0	0	0	2
Movement tracing	155	13	1	0	2	1
Cull sow serum survey	9	21	9	2	3	0
Communal boar survey	N/A**	N/A	1	3	0	0
Other farm serum survey	N/A	N/A	0	0	1	N/A
Reconfirmed in known infected herds	118	N/A	N/A	N/A	N/A	N/A
Totals	443	47	12	5	6	5

* to 31/5/88 only
**not applicable

EPIDEMIOLOGY

Epidemiology in a field situation is an inexact science fraught with many difficulties, particularly when studied within the constraints imposed by a stamping-out policy. Findings must always be viewed skeptically and interpreted with caution. The apparently obvious conclusion may often be incorrect. The discovery of considerable numbers of outbreaks in the course of carrying out 2 km patrols is not, per se, evidence of airborne spread of infection. The fact that disease was confirmed on a disproportionate number of premises on which waste food was fed may suggest waste food as a source of infection, but is actually an indication of the way British waste feeders purchase store pigs. Infected meat appears to play no part in the transmission of AD to pigs, and attempts to infect pigs by feeding tissues from pigs soon after challenge with field virus have been unsuccessful (Donaldson, *et al.*, 1984). Infection has been spread to dogs by this means however, probably through the medium of minced head meat sold for petfood.

An outbreak (ref DZ 340) in Lancashire in 1983 demonstrates the difficulty of attributing a correct origin. A fattening unit on which waste food was fed purchased store pigs at markets and from dealers. Fifty-five blood samples were collected on the farm on 8th June whilst tracing the movement of stores from another confirmed outbreak (DZ 187): all were negative. AD was subsequently confirmed serologically on a nearby premise (DZ 256), and a further 55 blood samples were collected on 13th July in the course of the 2 km patrol around DZ 256. This time 3 positives were found, all from pigs purchased in Preston Market on 15th June - after the previous sampling. The 2 vendors of the pigs making up the 37 purchased were traced: one was negative but 40 of 59 adults tested at the other were positive, and disease was confirmed. The true origin of DZ 340 was apparent partly because of a fortuitous combination of testing circumstances: area patrol sampling had identified an outbreak caused by the movement of store pigs from another, previously unknown, outbreak. Had the testing history been different the outbreak at DZ 340 could have attributed to pigs purchased from DZ 187 or, more tentatively, local spread from DZ 256.

The propensity shown by waste food feeders, in particular, for buying small numbers of stores from a large number of premises also made it difficult to know which infected breeding units had spread infection when selling stores. Twenty percent of the waste food feeders in Lancashire, the county with the largest number of such premises in Britain, were infected in 1983: when all tracings had been completed some were found to have purchased stores from 5 different infected breeding units and, whilst the source of infection was clearly purchased pigs, the attribution of responsibility to a specific vendor was rarely possible.

Other factors which made epidemiological study difficult included:

1. The rarity of clinical disease, in the absence of which it is difficult to establish when infection entered a herd. (Most outbreaks were diagnosed on serological evidence only).

2. The fact that many herds - particularly those investigated in Stage I -had been infected for long periods of time. Individual memory becomes fallible as time passes so that significant facts are forgotten.

3. Inability to recover AD virus from premises on which infection was longstanding. Attempts by colleagues at the Central Veterinary Laboratory, Weybridge, to recover virus by stressing seropositive pigs have been successful only when infection has been contracted within the preceding 12 months. DNA fingerprinting is potentially of particular value as an epidemiological tool when investigating outbreaks which are believed to be long-standing, but the technique cannot be utilised unless virus has been isolated.

Despite these reservations conclusions can be drawn.

A. Airborne spread

Experience during the eradication programme had produced little conclusive evidence for or against airborne spread of infection between farms. Many outbreaks were identified whilst carrying out 2 km patrols around infected premises but alternative explanations, such as the movement of pigs from other infected premises, were found in many cases: an example has already been described. Even in the absence of such pig movement the possible transfer of infection by movements of people or fomites can neither be proved nor disproved.

The best evidence for airborne spread of infection in Britain predates the start of eradication. A study of a series of outbreaks of AD in 11 herds in North Yorkshire in 1981-1982 suggested that airborne spread over distances considerably in excess of 2 km had occurred (Gloster *et al.*, 1984). The outbreaks exhibited a number of unusual features which had facilitated their study:

1. The date disease began in the area was readily established.
2. On the majority of farms the commencement of disease could be estimated within days.
3. The clinical symptoms of disease were marked.
4. On the majority of farms disease spread by other means, such as the movement of infected stock, could be eliminated, and routine tracings had failed to identify any other reason for disease spread.
5. The outbreaks were well documented.
6. Meteorological data were readily available from a nearby source.

The authors concluded that airborne transmission of infection was the possible cause of 7 of the 11 outbreaks. For each of the 7 a virus source was available coincident with the likely period of infection, and meteorological conditions were such that virus could have blown from the supposed source for many tens of hours. Contrary to the opinions of Bitsch and Andersen (1982), who believed that airborne disease transmission was possible for outbreaks separated by no more than 2 km, the maximum distance over which airborne spread was probably responsible for infection was 9 km. In the 2 outbreaks where airborne virus was believed to have travelled the greatest distances a combination of 2 events was recorded. Firstly, large quantities of virus would have been released into the atmosphere at the supposed source, and secondly, winds of a constant direction were present for many hours.

Despite this evidence the British control programme still utilises a 2 km patrol radius around infected farms as routine. We have no evidence to suggest that by doing so any outbreak has been missed, and certainly insufficient evidence to justify the massive increase in resources required to routinely blood sample herds in a larger area. An indication of the consequent increase is given by considering the number of pig herds within 2, 5 and 8 km of 4 confirmed outbreaks in Cheshire this year:

2 km patrol - average 5 herds (range 2 - 7)
5 km patrol - average 29 herds (range 28 - 30)
8 km patrol - average 66 herds (range 64 - 67)

The 2 km patrol radius is, however, increased in exceptional cases. This was done in 1983 in areas where confirmed outbreaks had been numerous and only limited areas remained outside the many 2 km patrols. Again, in Cheshire this spring a 4 mile (6 km) area was utilized around 2 outbreaks for which no origin was apparent, resulting in the discovery of 2 more outbreaks. Other links between the outbreaks were then established - knacker lorry and personnel movements, and shared equipment - so that airborne spread was no more than one of a number of possible methods by which infection had spread. On this occasion the patrol area was extended yet further to sample every pig within 8 km of any of the outbreaks, but the exercise did not disclose any more infected herds.

B. Movements of infected pigs

According to McFerran (1981) infection usually gains entry to a pig farm by the introduction of a subclinically infected pig. Our experience has been that the sale of pigs during and shortly after clinical outbreaks is the most important method of spread, whilst breeding movements of sows to boars or boars to sows also play a significant role.

We have observed considerable variation between one infected breeding unit and another in their apparent ability to disseminate infection by selling store pigs, even when no clinical disease is apparent on the breeding unit. The majority do not, in fact, spread infection. At one non-clinical outbreak in 1987, 42 of 58 adults sampled were positive at the diagnostic blood sampling, some at very high titers. In the 22 weeks preceding confirmation 1081 store pigs had been moved to one fattening unit. No serological evidence of infection was found on this fattening unit, or on 11 others to which fewer pigs had been sent. Such a finding has not been uncommon: we have tested many fattening units and found no seropositive pigs although every pig on that fattening unit had been obtained from an infected breeding unit. Seropositive pigs may, however, be found when testing suckling or recently weaned piglets on such breeding units: in the example quoted 9/10 suckling and 4/40 recently weaned pigs were positive, the former at higher titres than the latter. These titres presumably reflect passive immunity derived from maternal colostrum, rather than active infection.

A few non-clinical breeding units do, however, spread infection. An example studied in Lancashire in 1983 involved a breeding herd in which 40 of the 59 adults sampled were positive but with no history of clinical disease. Tracing 23 farms to which store pigs had been sold disclosed 8 more outbreaks and, in addition, pigs had been sold to 4 other farms on which disease had already been confirmed in the course of other tracings. In my experience the feature that distinguishes herds which continue to spread infection when clinical disease is not present from those which do not is the standard of management: where conditions are poor and stock under continual stress infection is likely to be spread.

C. Communal boars

The importance of communal boars in spreading AD had not been appreciated prior to the start of the eradication programme, but quickly became apparent in Lancashire, North Wales and the West Country. Communal boars are not a common feature of British pig farming practice, and the farms with which they are involved are mostly small. One such enterprise owned 4 boars, 3 of which were seropositive when sampled in 1983. Breeding movements had taken place to and from 15 other farms, a boar sometimes travelling to serve a sow and, in other cases, the sow visiting the communal boar unit. AD was subsequently confirmed on serological evidence on 8 of the 15 farms traced. The premises infected included farms to which the boar had been sent as well as farms which had sent sows to the boar.

LATENCY

There is no doubt that breeding units in which infection is asymptomatic may, in certain circumstances, spread infection by selling store pigs. It is questionable whether infection is truly latent in pigs on these premises or on the more numerous examples which are not responsible for spread, since study of the age distribution of seropositive pigs, and the serological titres of purchased replacement breeding stock (such as boars) usually indicates continuing spread of infection amongst adult pigs. If we regard latency as the reactivation of a truly quiescent infection, evidence that this has occurred in the field in Great Britain is very limited. Experience indicates that in the majority of cases latent infection is not reactivated: only occasional cases suggest the contrary.

In this context the series of outbreaks confirmed earlier this year in North-West England and North Wales is of particular interest, although the evidence is limited by our inability to recover virus from sows believed to have been infected more than 12 months before. The outbreak details are listed in Table 3 and the methods by which infection spread illustrated diagrammatically in Fig. 2.

TABLE 3 Details of outbreaks confirmed in 1988 (to 31/5)

Herd[1] Ref.	Herd[2] Type	Stock details and test results												Date clinical signs first seen	Virus isolation
		Boars			Sows + Gilts			Weaned			Suckling				
		a	b	c	a	b	c	a	b	c	a	b	c		
A	B/F	7	7	4	144	51	47	1200	31	28	222	0	—	1/88	+
B	B/F	10	8	5	210	56	52	967	25	22	100	0	—	11/87	+
C	F	0	—	—	0	—	—	1341	58	32	0	—	—	N/A	
D	B/F	5	5	2	117	32	29	620	11	0	160	0	—	6/87	—
E	W/B	2	2	2	34	34	27	113	53	0	97	12	5	N/A	—
F	F	0	—	—	0	—	—	1076	483	14	0	—	—	N/A	+

1. a = total, b = sampled, c = positive. Herds ref A-E were confirmed and slaughtered.
2. Herd ref F was not confirmed, but seropositive pigs were slaughtered.

B/F = Breeder/Fattener
W/B = Weaner/Breeder
F = Fattener

AD virus was recovered from post mortem material from farms A and B, on both of which acute clinical disease was seen, and by stressing seropositive pigs from farm F. Attempts to recover virus from seropositive sows on farms D and E were unsuccessful, and isolation was not attempted from farm C. DNA fingerprinting confirmed that apparently identical viruses had caused outbreaks on A, B and F (and, by inference, on D). The virus fingerprints closely resembled those of viruses isolated in Britain in 1982 and 1983, before the start of the eradication programme. It would have been invaluable if virus could have been recovered from farm E since fingerprinting could have confirmed the supposition that this outbreak was the origin of the series: even without that evidence we believe this to have been the case.

The Welsh breeding unit, farm E, practiced an unusual form of management. Sows and boars were kept to a great age, and the only pig moved to the farm in the 7 years before disease was confirmed was a replacement boar which had been purchased in May 1986. The vendors premises were traced and sampled, and no evidence of infection was found but the boar had been seropositive at the diagnostic bleed at farm E in February 1988 - indicating that infection had been contracted after arrival on the premises.

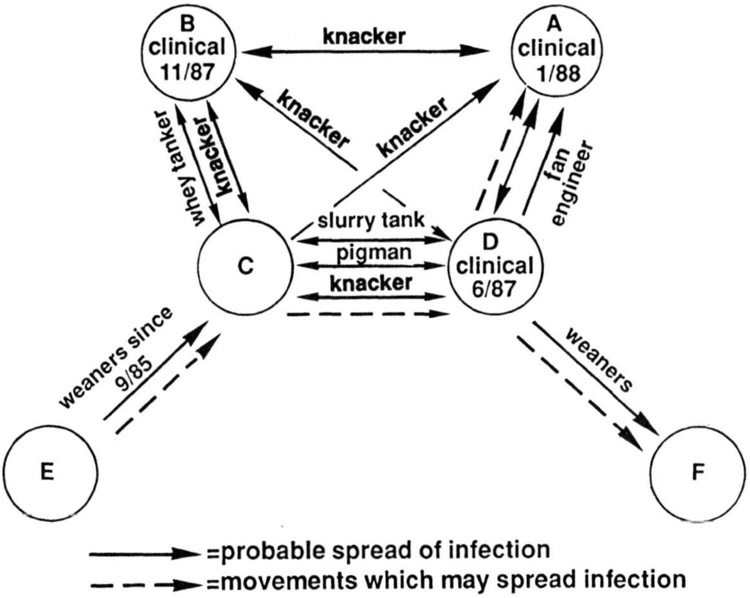

Fig. 2 1988 outbreaks - diagrammatic representation.

Twenty-five of 32 adult breeding pigs on farm E were positive when diagnostic sampling (as a possible origin for the outbreak on farm C) was carried out. Fifteen weaned pigs were also included in the diagnostic sampling, but all were negative. Blood samples were subsequently collected from 38 weaned and 12 suckling pigs before slaughter: all weaned pigs were negative, but 5 of the suckling piglets were seropositive.

Since April 1986 all 730 weaners produced had been sold to farm C, but before that date 14 other farms had been supplied. All 14 were traced and were negative. It is our opinion that infection must have been present, asymptomatic and unrecognized, for many years. This may, therefore be an example of the reactivation of a latent infection, although careful investigation has failed to identify any reason for such reactivation on the breeding unit. It may be significant, however, that farm C suffered a severe outbreak of swine dysentery in 1987, during which more than 300 pigs died. The stress which surviving pigs suffered at this time may, perhaps, have been the trigger factor on the fattening unit which reactivated latent virus in one or more of the weaners purchased from farm E.

REFERENCES

Agriculture, Fisheries and Food. Ministry of. 1984. "Animal Health 1983: Report of the Chief Veterinary Officer". (HMSO. London) p. 10.

Bitsch, V. and Andersen, J.B. 1982. On the epidemiology of Aujeszky's disease in Denmark and the possibilities of its control. Curr. Top. Vet. Anim. Sci., **17,** 227-236. In: CEC Seminar on "Aujeszky's Disease". (Eds. G. Wittmann and S.A. Hall). (Martinus Nijhoff, The Hague).

Donaldson, A.I., Wardley, R.C., Martin, S. and Harkness, J.W. 1984. Influence of vaccination on Aujeszky's disease virus and disease transmission, Vet. Rec., **115,** 121-124.

Gloster, J., Donaldson, A.I. and Hough, M.N. 1984. Analysis of a series of outbreaks of Aujeszky's disease in Yorkshire 1981-1982: The possibility of airborne disease spread. Vet. Rec., **114,** 234-239.

McFerran, J.B. 1981. Proceedings of the Pig Veterinary Society, **8,** 44.

CURRENT THINKING ON THE ROLE OF VACCINES IN ERADICATION STRATEGIES FOR AUJESZKY'S DISEASE IN THE USA

D.G. Thawley, R. Morrison

University of Minnesota, College of Veterinary Medicine
Large Animal Clinical Sciences, 225 Veterinary Teaching Hospitals
1365 Gortner Avenue, St. Paul, MN 55108

ABSTRACT

Since 1974, the prevalence of Aujeszky's disease within the United States has increased more than 15 fold. As a result, in 1987, a national eradication program was proposed and has been supported by the National Pork Producer's Council. Several strategies for eradicating Aujeszky's disease from herds of swine have been evaluated and proven successful. The appropriate use of vaccine is considered highly beneficial in many control and eradication programs for Aujeszky's disease. The ability to differentiate pigs which have been vaccinated from infected pigs is crucial to the further refinement of control programs.

INTRODUCTION

The United States has a long history of Aujeszky's disease (AD). In 1813 a case of "mad-itch" was reported in Ohio. This was 89 years before Dr. Aladar Aujeszky described classical AD. Later in 1931, Dr. R.E. Shope demonstrated that "mad-itch" and AD were identical. Until 1960, the disease in swine was mild and very rare. In the early 1970's the prevalence of AD increased. Serological surveys conducted by the United States Federal Government indicated a prevalence of infection of 0.56% in 1974. This increased to 3.73% in 1978 to 8.39% in 1981 and 8.78% by 1984 (Schnurrenberger, 1984).

Within the United States, initial concern about the increasing prevalence of AD resulted in a federally sponsored fact-finding conference in 1977[1]. In May 1979, new federal regulations were put into place which required serological testing of all breeding stock prior to interstate movement. All herds which contained AD-positive animals were quarantined with stock movement to slaughter only.

Between 1977-1983 a number of studies were conducted to investigate various

[1] Proceedings, Pseudorabies Fact-Finding Conference. April 4-5, 1977.

J. T. van Oirschot (ed.), Vaccination and Control of Aujeszky's Disease, 197–208.

strategies to clear herds of AD-positive animals (Wright *et al.*, 1982). In 1983 these studies culminated in a 5-state project called the "PRV Pilot Projects" which was a large scale effort to investigate the feasibility of eradicating AD on an area-wide basis. The final report noted that eradication was feasible, and the authors strongly recommended these efforts be conducted on an area-wide basis (Thawley *et al.*, 1987). The report also concluded that: "the provision of vaccine by government stimulated participation. The use of vaccination was compatible with herd clean-up plans".

In late 1986 and early 1987 an eradication program was drafted by the Livestock Conservation Institute and the U.S. Animal Health Association. In March 1987 this plan was supported by 87% of the delegates to the Natural Pork Producers Council at the Pork Congress in Indianapolis. This plan, which remains in draft form, calls for a phased introduction of nationwide eradication program which would initially be organized at the level of individual states. The eradication program has 5 proposed phases:

Stage 1: Preparation.

To qualify for Stage 1, a State Aujeszky's Disease Committee must be formed and plans formulated for a reliable system of determining the prevalence of AD in the state swine population and reports submitted to the Federal Government.

Stage 2: Control.

In this stage a state commits itself to eradication. Its goals are to determine which herds are infected and to begin eradication programs within infected herds.

Stage 3: Mandatory Herd Clean-up.

In this stage, all infected herds must begin eradication plans.

Stage 4: Surveillance.

To enter Stage 4, a state must have had a surveillance program in place for at least 2 years and no new cases of AD may have occurred in the previous 12 months. The surveillance program must utilize the testing of marketed cull breeding stock.

Stage 5: Aujeszky's Disease Free.

This is the stage in which a state will be declared free of AD. The state must have been free of AD for a minimum of 1 year.

CURRENT STATE ORGANIZED PROGRAMS

In the late 1970's several states initiated programs to certify breeding herds which were free of pseudorabies virus (PRV). Certification was formalized by the introduction of the qualified PRV-free states initiated by the Federal Government in

1979. To be rated qualified PRV-free, the entire breeding herd must be initially tested AD-seronegative. To maintain qualified free status 25% of the breeding herd must be retested every 3 months, or 10% tested every month.

In 1985 the state of Illinois introduced a rule that prohibited the movement of feeder pigs into or within Illinois unless they originate from a qualified PRV-free herd or from a herd which is tested annually (a random sample of approximately 30 breeding swine per herd). Many states are now introducing similar rules for feeder pig movement. In addition, several states are drafting plans for full eradication programs which will utilize either the systematic testing of all herds, or blood testing of slaughter sows and boars. These plans are being coordinated to meet the guidelines of the national eradication program currently in review.

STRATEGIES FOR ERADICATING AD FROM HERDS OF SWINE

Swine herds and/or premises can be freed of PRV. When AD is diagnosed in a herd, all factors must be considered, a plan chosen and rigidly adhered to. Alterations to a basic plan can be made to take advantage of the particular premise; however, the basic principles must be scrupulously followed. Three basic clean-up strategies have been previously described (Thawley et al., 1982). These include:

- Test and Removal of positive animals. This procedure rebuilds a herd from seronegative adults;
- Offspring Segregation followed by Phased Repopulation of Herd;
- Depopulation / Repopulation.

Vaccination programs are often important components of these plans.

Preliminary considerations in deciding how to proceed should include:

- Evaluation of laboratory data and, if necessary, reconfirmation of the diagnosis;
- Consideration of the vaccination status of the herd;
- Consideration of type of management, housing, size of breeding herd, other domestic animals with direct contact with pigs, personnel and vehicle traffic, herd additions and source of replacements, presence of wild animals, dead animal disposal;
- Consideration of the prevalence of PRV in the neighborhood.

Within most herds, PRV must be removed from 2 populations of pigs:

the breeding herd, and the growing/finishing operation. Large herds which are PRV-seropositive are more frequently infected in both the breeding and growing/finishing herds than smaller herds which are frequently infected in only the breeding herd.

An initial step in clean-up is to identify by serologic testing the prevalence of infection, where PRV-seropositive animals reside in the herd, the ages of animals infected, etc.

- Breeding Herd

  Blood test 30 breeding sows, gilts and boars.

- Growing/Finishing Herd

  A representative sample of finishing pigs (16+ weeks) must be tested. A minimum sample includes 30 pigs per building which have been randomly selected from all pens. Record the age and location of each pig bled. Based on blood test results, a strategy is selected which is directed toward clearing the herd of PRV infection. Following the initial sampling of the breeding and finishing herds, a plan must be made which will provide the most cost effective means to clear the herd of PRV infection. Details of plans are described below.

STRATEGIES TO REMOVE PRV FROM THE BREEDING HERD

1. Test and Removal

Under favorable conditions, this option may be least disruptive to management and is least costly. In some herds it may be combined with an early vaccination program. It probably will not be successful in a herd with total confinement and all ages in a single building with a common ventilation system. It should not be attempted in a herd in such a confinement system, or in herds with current clinical signs or evidence of continuing spread. The lower the prevalence, the more likely it is to succeed. Three options are available:

1(a) Test and Removal without Vaccination

Use this option when less than 20-25% of the breeding herd is PRV-seropositive and there is no evidence of infection in the growing or finishing pens.

Test the entire breeding herd every 30 days and remove all seropositive swine. All seropositive swine must be considered potential sources of infection. If, after 3 tests, seropositive animals continue to be found in the herd, this method should be re-evaluated. Positive animals must be moved immediately to slaughter or to a quarantined feeding facility.

Following one negative test, the herd may be considered free of PRV.

1(b) Vaccination followed by Test and Removal

This option may be used when a high percentage of the breeding herd is seropositive and/or there is evidence of infection in growing or finishing pens. Test all breeding animals and identify PRV-seropositive ones. Vaccinate the entire breeding herd with a killed PRV vaccine at 6 month intervals. Recently developed vaccines which allow the differentiation of vaccinated from infected pigs may also be used. Rotate out all original PRV-seropositive sows. Six months after the last vaccination, (immediately if differentiable vaccines have been used) test all breeding animals and a representative sample of offspring over 16 weeks of age. If the offspring test negative, remove all positive sows and retest as in 1(a).

1(c) Phased Test and Removal with Vaccination

To minimize the interruption to pig flow, a phased test and removal plan may be used. Inherent in this plan is increased risk of failure to eliminate PRV from the herd because positive pigs remain in the herd for longer periods of time. However, the risk may be reduced by vaccination and may be more than offset by the reduced cost of the program. All sows and boars are tested and then vaccinated with a killed or differentiable vaccine to enhance their immunity and lessen the risk of virus spread until all the originally positive sows are removed from the herd at their next weaning. All positive boars are immediately removed from the herd. Positive sows are replaced after weaning with unvaccinated or vaccinated gilts. Stop vaccination after all original positives are removed. Four to 6 months after vaccination, (immediately, if differentiable vaccines have been used) all sows are tested and any remaining positives are immediately removed from the herd. Retest herd in 30 days and continue to monitor as in Option 1(a). This method is often the most cost effective procedure to use in large herds as it causes minimal production losses in the herd and does not interrupt pig flow in the operation.

2. Offspring Segregation followed by Total Replacement of the Breeding Herd (With or Without Vaccination).

A strategy of offspring segregation is being utilized to produce PRV-seronegative gilt replacements from positive sow herds. This allows genetic material to be salvaged from valuable breeding herds. In this procedure the offspring of PRV-seropositive sows are raised in segregated facilities. Salvaging of offspring is effective because pigs nursing immune sows receive a considerable level of protection against clinical disease. After the first 24 hours, the pig's antibody level declines on a half-life basis and is no longer detectable in most pigs by 12 weeks of age, but may persist to 16 weeks in some pigs (Gustafson, 1986). Maternal antibody levels in pigs from naturally infected sows are usually higher and persist longer than from vaccinated, uninfected dams, with even higher titers from infected dams which have been vaccinated prior to farrowing. It is desired that colostral antibody protection be as high and as widespread as possible in the piglets in the farrowing house. Pigs from selected females are weaned at 3-4 weeks of age, or as early as possible. Replacement gilts which will become the foundation of a new herd are selected and moved to segregated facilities. Pigs can be moved to the negative herd over a period of time, but the longer the period and the more pigs moved, the greater the chance of transmission of the virus to the uninfected herd. All isolated gilts are tested at 16 weeks of age. Maternal antibodies should be gone, resulting in negative serological findings. All seropositive gilts must be considered potential sources of infection and removed. If any pigs in a pen test positive, all pigs in the pen should be immediately removed from the segregated herd. As entire pens test negative, they can be combined into larger units to eventually establish the new herd. The breeding herd should be vaccinated prior to beginning the offspring segregation program, and should receive booster vaccinations at appropriate intervals until all original stock have been replaced.

Breed the segregated gilts to new, uninfected boars and hold in segregation through gestation. These bred animals may be vaccinated or remain unvaccinated and then be introduced into the breeding herd as replacements in a total herd replacement program. Alternatively, segregated gilts may be used as replacements in a "test and removal" program.

3. Depopulation / Repopulation

This option is only recommended as a last resort. It is the plan most likely to succeed, but may be only necessary in confinement operations with high prevalence of infection. This option is more viable if any of the following apply in the herd:

- A high percentage of seropositives (over 80% of breeding animals) indicates that PRV is spreading, especially if there is an increasing prevalence or appearance of new seropositive pigs in repeated tests.
- Genetic strains have little value.
- There are multiple disease problems in the herd.
- The herd is housed in confinement with a common air source or where separation is difficult to maintain.

A significant advantage of this choice is the opportunity to repopulate with healthier, genetically superior swine. Other diseases may be causing as much, or more, loss as AD. Replacement animals may be vaccinated with a differentiable vaccine and monitored accordingly.

STRATEGIES TO REMOVE PRV FROM THE GROWING / FINISHING HERD

In cases where breeding herds are infected with PRV, the infection is often found to circulate within the growing/finishing animals. To free the herd of PRV it is therefore necessary to stop the circulation of virus within the grower/finishers. Once this is achieved the natural flow of pigs through the facility will free the grower/finisher operation of PRV within 3-5 months.

Strategies for stopping circulation of PRV within the growing/finishing pigs are currently being investigated. It is recognized that in most herds evidence of virus circulation exists only in pigs of 14 weeks and older. Most likely, maternally derived antibodies retard circulation until pigs enter the late growing stage. Therefore, the principle means of preventing circulation of virus is to actively stimulate an immune response in pigs to provide protection until marketing. At present the best method to achieve this is by vaccinating growing fattening pigs when maternal antibody levels are reduced sufficiently to permit a response to vaccination. Optimally, 10 pigs in each 10, 12, 14, 16, 18, 20 and 22 week age groups should be blood tested. From the test results, it may be determined at what age transmission begins to occur in the growing/fattening pigs. A recent study of 15 herds in Minnesota found that 3 basic types of serological profiles are observed in growing/finishing pigs on infected farms (Fig. 1). In the "negative" herd, the prevalence of positive pigs declined from approximately 8 to 12 weeks of age. No positive pigs were detected after this age. In the "high-positive" profile, the prevalence of positive pigs declined from 8 to 12 weeks of age and then increased such that approximately 100% were positive by 18 to 26 weeks of age. A profile called "low-positive" was observed as an intermediate stage between "high-positive" and "negative" in several herds. The prevalence declined similar to other profiles, but there were several negative groups of pigs from 12 to 18 weeks of age before positive groups were detected. Four of the 15 herds that started "negative" remained "negative" for the duration of the study. Four of the "high-positive" herds remained "high-positive" throughout the study. Four herds became "negative" and reverted to "high-positive". In some herds, it appears as though the spread of PRV within the growing/finishing herd stops abruptly and the virus is eliminated from this section as the infected pigs are sold. The use of cross sectional serological profiles of pigs from 8-26 weeks of age was helpful in determining if PRV was actively spreading in this section of the herd.

It is thought that vaccination of growing pigs may prevent the spread of field virus which results in the "high-positive" and "low-positive" profiles. A vaccination program should then be initiated in which pigs are vaccinated 3 weeks prior to this determined age. If this age cannot be determined it is best to vaccinate pigs twice; once as they leave the nursery and again at 12-14 weeks of age. During the period when PRV-seropositive pigs are in the growing/finishing facilities, replacement breeding stock must be selected from outside sources or from an identified source of PRV-seronegative gilts on the farm. Once all PRV-seropositive animals are removed, an on-farm source of replacement may be used.

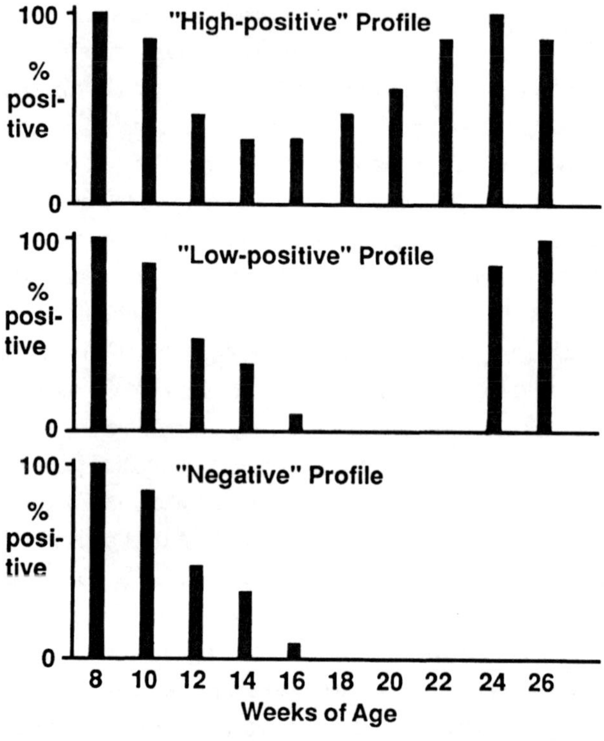

Fig. 1 Serological profiles for PRV observed in cross sectional growing/finishing section of herds.

ROLE OF VACCINES

Several vaccines against AD are currently being used in the United States (Molitor and Thawley, 1987). The major vaccines are listed in Table 1.

TABLE 1 Major AD virus vaccines in the USA

Vaccine	Company	Original Strain	Gene Deletion
Modified Live Virus Vaccines			
PR-Vac	Norden Laboratories	BUK	gI
Pseudorabies Vaccine	Bio-Ceutic Laboratories	Bartha	gI
Pseudovax	Pitman-Moore	BUK	Unknown
Omnivac-PRV-1	Fermenta	BUK	TK
Omnivac-PRV-2	Fermenta	BUK	TK and gIII
PRV-Marker	Syntrovet	Iowa	TK and gX, repeat region deletion and gene insertion
Tolvid	Upjohn	Aujeszky's strain	TK and gX
Killed Virus Vaccines			
Pr-VaC-Killed	Norden Laboratories		
Suvaxyn-PRV	Solvay Veterinary		
Porci-Rab	Beecham Laboratories		

Over the past several years the use of vaccines has gained increasing acceptance in strategies designed to control and eradicate AD. Their use is based on several assumptions:

1. Vaccinated herds have less clinical outbreaks if infected.
2. Pigs from vaccinated sows will usually have adequate antibody against PRV until 8-12 weeks of age.
3. It takes a higher dose of virus to infect a vaccinated animal than an unvaccinated animal.
4. Vaccination against AD reduces losses from other infections such as hemophilus pneumonia, etc.
5. Differential tests will be available to distinguish between antibodies produced by vaccine and those produced by field viruses.
6. Modified live vaccines given to a negative animal will elicit a more complete immunological response which will be of longer duration than that produced by a killed vaccine.
7. The use of vaccines is more likely to gain the cooperation of herd owners.

Several of our own research studies indicate that appropriate use of vaccines may facilitate the removal of virus from a herd. We suggest that an appropriate vaccination program may reduce or prevent the spread of virus within a herd by reducing the level of recrudescence and increasing the resistance of individual pigs to infection.

We consider the larger the herd, the greater the probability that in any given time period, virus recrudescence will occur in the herd. The probability of recrudescence of infection occurring in a herd is proportional to the size of the herd, the percentage of the herd which is PRV-seropositive due to infection with field virus, the probability of a single pig becoming recrudescent, and the length of time latent carriers remain in the herd. This may be represented by the following formula:

$$P = (N) \times (W) \times (T) \times (K)$$

where

P = probabilitiy of recrudescence within herd
N = herd size
W = prevalence of PRV positive pigs (due to infection with field virus)
T = average time PRV positive pigs (due to infection with field virus) remain in herd
K = probability of recrudescence in a single PRV positive pig

This equation explains why large herds have a greater probability of experiencing recrudescence of infection. Considering the formula, recrudescence within a herd may be minimized by:

- Reducing (W) and (T), the prevalence of PRV-seropositive pigs and the average time that PRV-seropositive pigs remain in the herd. This may be achieved by replacing PRV-seropositive pigs as rapidly as possible during the clean-up process.
- Reducing (K), the probability of recrudescence in a single PRV-seropositive pig. Management may play an important role in reducing the possibility of recrudescence in a single pig. Immune stimulation via vaccination may suppress recrudescence of latent carriers. Therefore, a vaccination program may significantly reduce the probability of recrudescence within the herd, particularly in cases where PRV-seropositive pigs will remain in the herd for extended periods. Since recrudescence may also be stimulated by stress, efforts should be taken to minimize stresses caused by management, such as the movement and mixing of pigs, change in environmental temperature, density, etc.
- Reducing N, herd size, will reduce the risk of recrudescence and transmission during the clean-up period.

Vaccination trials which have been conducted in growing pigs on 4 farms compared the effect that type of vaccine had on subsequent weight gain (Table 2). When data from all farms were analyzed together, there was a significant farm effect ($p<0.001$) on weight gain. Pigs with or without antibody at initial selection subsequently gained 146.2 and 125.8 pounds, respectively ($p<0.005$). Vaccine type had no significant effect ($p<0.100$) on weight gain. When data from each farm were analyzed separately, vaccinated pigs at one farm gained approximately 4 kg more from 8 to 23 weeks of age ($p<0.10$). No benefit was observed at the other farms. The variable effect of vaccine on weight gain may be due to differences between PRV strains since some strains have been reported to be more virulent than others. Farm characteristics such as management and building design, genetics, and concurrent diseases may also play a role in determining the effect of PRV infection on weight gain.

In general, the appropriate use of vaccine is considered highly beneficial in many control and eradication programs for AD. The ability to differentiate pigs which have been vaccinated from infected pigs is crucial to the further refinement of control programs. The rapid introduction and validation of vaccines and diagnostic tests which will permit differentiation is being keenly monitored.

TABLE 2 Weight gain (pounds) observed in growing pigs from 8-22 weeks of age following PRV vaccination.

Vaccine	Farm 1		Farm 2	Farm 3	Farm 4
	Pilot 1	Pilot 2			
No vaccine	128^{ab}	178^{c}	118^{c}	124^{a}	169^{a}
KV 1x IM	133^{a}	nd	130^{d}	123_{a}	170^{a}
KV 1x IP	121^{b}	nd	nd	nd	nd
KV 2x IM	nd	173^{a}	133^{d}	116^{a}	163^{a}
MLV 1x IM	119^{b}	nd	126^{cd}	126^{a}	169^{a}
MLV 2x IM	nd	167^{a}	nd	nd	nd

^{ab} different superscripts denote difference ($p<0.05$).
^{cd} different superscripts denote difference ($p<0.10$).
1x = 1 dose; 2x = 2 doses given 2 weeks apart.
nd = not done.
IP = intraperitoneally; IM = intramuscularly

REFERENCES

Gustafson, D.F. 1986. Pseudorabies. In: Diseases of Swine. 6th Ed., (Eds. A.D. Leman, B. Straw, R. Glock, W.L. Mengeling, R.H.C. Penny and E. Schnoll). (Iowa State University Press, Ames, Iowa). pp. 274-289.

Molitor, T. and Thawley, D.G. 1987. Pseudorabies Vaccines, Past, Present and Future. Compendium Food Animal, **9,** 409-416.

Proceedings, Pseudorabies Fact-Finding Conference. April 4-5, 1977.

Schnurrenberger, L.W. 1984. Slaughter Serum Surveys. Proceeding Livestock Conservation Institute. pp. 170-171.

Thawley, D.G., Beran, G.W., Hogg, A., Gustafson, D. and Vinson, R. 1987. Summary Report of the Pseudorabies Pilot Projects. J. Am. Vet. Med. Assn., **191,** 1386-1390.

Thawley, D.G., Gustafson, D.P. and Beran, G.W. 1982. Procedures for the Elimination of Pseudorabies Virus from Herds of Swine. J. Am. Vet. Med. Assn., **181,** 1513-1518.

Wright, J.C., Thawley, D.G. and Solerzano, R.F. 1982. Field evaluation of test and removal and vaccination as control measures for pseudorabies in Missouri swine. Can. J. Comp. Med., **46,** 420-425.

PRESENT AND FUTURE CONTROL OF AUJESZKY'S DISEASE IN THE FEDERAL REPUBLIC OF GERMANY

G. Wittmann

Federal Center for Virus Diseases of Animals,
PO Box 1149, D-7400 Tübingen, FRG

ABSTRACT

Despite the implementation of measures to control Aujeszky's disease, the virus continued to spread. Plans for future control include mass vaccination with glycoprotein I deleted vaccines in conjunction with serological testing and culling of infected sows. The cost for a 6-year eradication program is estimated to be approximately DM 500 million.

PRESENT CONTROL

Until 1977, only between 2 and 24 Aujeszky's disease (AD) outbreaks in pigs were recorded in the Federal Republic of Germany (FRG) per year. From 1977 onwards, their number has increased, reaching 1968 outbreaks in 1987 (see Fig. 1). However, this does not reflect the real figure since a considerable number of outbreaks may not have been reported by the farmers to avoid restrictions.

The outbreaks are concentrated in regions with dense pig populations in Northern and North-west Germany. Fattening herds are most frequently affected. However, since 1986 an increasing tendency is noticed in Bavaria (173 outbreaks in 1987). Therefore, there is a risk that the disease will spread to other pig centers in Southern Germany, especially to Baden-Württenberg and Hesse, where 13 and 29 outbreaks, respectively, were recorded in spring 1988.

Besides pigs, cattle are affected more and more with occasional recoveries. A link to infected pigs could not be detected in all instances.

Legislative measures, including duty of notification, have been ordered in herds with clinical AD since 1980: killing of all the clinically affected pigs and all the suckling piglets in a herd to reduce the amount of shedded virus, vaccination, removal of pigs only for slaughter, thermotreatment of meat and offal, destruction of dead animals, aborted fetuses, stillborn piglets and afterbirths, non-use of semen for artificial insemination, disinfestation of rats, decontamination of dung, liquid manure and waste material, disinfection of implements, vehicles and of thoroughfares in the

J. T. van Oirschot (ed.), Vaccination and Control of Aujeszky's Disease, 209–213.

stable, including entrance and exit of the pig-shed. Unauthorized persons, cats and dogs must be kept away from the pig-shed. Authorized persons have to decontaminate and disinfect their hands, clothing and shoes, when leaving the shed.

Initially the ban was lifted when all the pigs were removed or the offspring of vaccinated pigs became seronegative. However, this resulted in overpopulation. Therefore, this restriction was relieved in 1982. Depending on the maximal period of virus excretion and incubation time, the ban is now lifted when 35 days have elapsed from the last clinical case of AD in a vaccinated herd. However, after this time pigs can only be removed for slaughter or for transfer into a vaccinated herd. All vaccinated animals are marked.

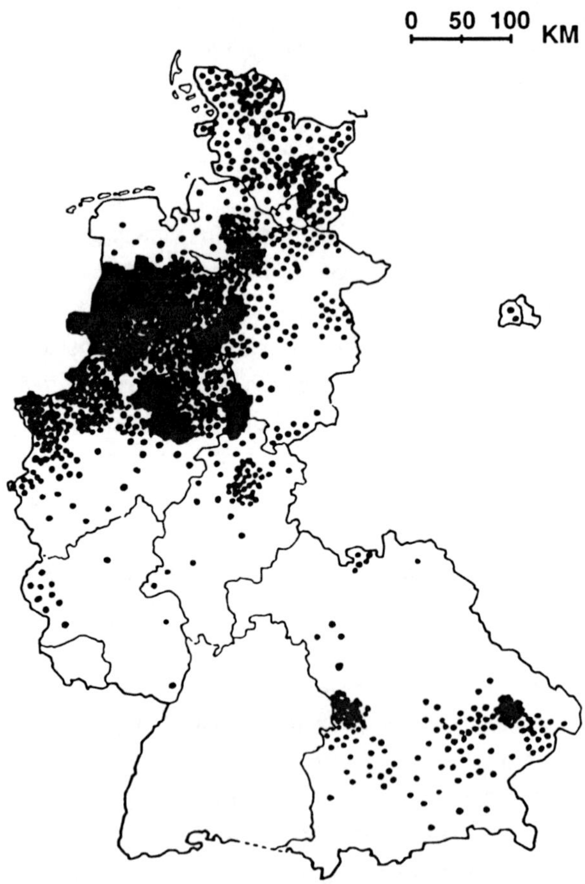

Fig. 1 Distribution of Aujeszky's disease outbreaks in the Federal Republic of Germany in 1987 (1968 outbreaks).

In some Federal States quarantine and serological examination of imported pigs is compulsory.

From 1980 to 1982 about DM 61.0 million were paid for compensation for killed pigs. Nevertheless, the disease spreads further. This is not surprising since the partially depopulated and vaccinated herds remain latently infected. Therefore, partial killing was abandoned in the heavily infected districts, where only vaccination is being practiced now. Slaughter of the whole infected herd is only practiced with single isolated outbreaks in non-infected districts.

PLANS FOR FUTURE CONTROL

The present situation of AD is rather hopeless in some regions of Germany. Therefore an expert committee was established in 1987, to make proposals for an efficient control and eradication of AD in Germany. I want to report on the preliminary plan.

The newly developed vaccine strains with gene deletions allow the differentiation between field virus-infected and vaccinated animals. Therefore, it seems promising to perform prophylactic vaccination on a large scale in infected areas and to eliminate the latently infected pigs. As a first step, the use of live vaccines will be allowed in the FRG this year. However, their use will be restricted to non-breeding herds. Breeding herds must be vaccinated with inactivated vaccines, as in the past. Only virus strains with deletion of the gene encoding glycoprotein I (gI) will be admitted for live and inactivated vaccines. We know that any other deletion can be used for differentiating field virus-infected pigs and vaccinated pigs. However, certain reasons are in favor of using the same deleted virus throughout the country:

(a) to avoid the potential risk of virulent recombinations between vaccine strains with different deletions,

(b) to avoid that laboratories have to use several ELISA kits and

(c) to be in accordance with The Netherlands in which only gI-deleted vaccines will be permitted, at least for breeding pigs. The narrow trade relations between the 2 countries do necessitate this.

Pigs vaccinated with live vaccines are not allowed to be removed from the herd during 21 days after vaccination. This shall prevent infections of dogs and cats by meat and offal, since the vaccine strains possess some residual virulence for carnivores. Mass vaccination is to be performed for 3 years until the sanitation program will begin. We hope that the amount of circulating field virus will be considerably reduced during this time. Fattening pig herds should be vaccinated once per fattening period. We are aware that this procedure does not evoke optimal immunity, however, the costs for 2 vaccinations would be too high. Breeding pigs should be vaccinated 3 times a year. The vaccination program should run for 6 years. The sanitation program will begin 3 years after the initiation of the vaccination program. Breeding pigs should be serologically examined twice a year. In parallel, all gI-seropositive breeding pigs should be slaughtered. No sanitation program including serological survey is provided for vaccinated fattening herds. Vaccination is supposed to diminish virus spread in the herds and finally cause the disappearance of virus.

What about the estimated costs? They are as yet available for 2 Federal States, Lower Saxony and North-Rhine-Westphalia (Table 1). These states produce 60% of the German pigs and have 79% of the AD outbreaks (1567 in 1987).

Vaccination of 26.5 million pigs affords DM 20.1 million for vaccines and DM 23.7 million for the veterinarians. That means in total DM 43.8 million per year and DM 262.8 million for 6 years.

TABLE 1 Estimated costs of the eradication program in 2 Federal States, which produce 60% of the German pigs and have 79% of the AD outbreaks (1567 in 1987)

Year		DM / million
1	Vaccination*	43.8**
2	Vaccination	43.8**
3	Vaccination	43.8**
4	Vaccination	43.8**
	Serolog. testing (sows)	24.4
	Compensation (76.000 sows)	38.0
5	Vaccination	43.8**
	Serolog. testing (sows)	24.4
	Compensation (15.360 sows)	6.1
6	Vaccination	43.8**
	Serolog. testing (sows)	24.4
	Compensation (15.360 sows)	6.1
		386.2
Other Federal States		~116.0 ?
		502.2

* Breeding sows (4.6 million) are vaccinated 3 times, and fattening pigs (25 million) are vaccinated once

** Inclusive DM 23.7 million for veterinarians

The serological survey in 1.54 million breeding sows, that are 3.1 million single tests, costs DM 24.4 million per year and DM 73.2 million in 3 years (year 4 to 6). The slaughter of seropositive sows, estimated 5% in year 4, 1% in year 5 and 6, respectively, should be subsidized by DM 38.0 million in year 4 and DM 6.1 million in year 5 and 6. In total DM 50.2 million. The total costs of the eradication program amount in total to DM 386.2 million for the 2 most heavily infected Federal States.

Data on the other Federal States, which produce about 40% of the German pigs, will be available in a few weeks. The incidence of AD in these States is about 21% of the total outbreaks. Therefore, I guess that vaccination will cost DM 66.0 million, serological testing DM 37.0 million and compensation DM 13.0 million. In total DM 116 million. Thus the 6-year eradication program may cost about DM 502.2 million in the FRG. About 50% of this amount of money should be paid by the insurance cooperations of the farmers. It is questionable if they are able to do this, since the income of the pig farmers is as low as 20 years ago and they may be not willing to undergo this additional burden.

For the initiation of the program we have to guarantee that it will work. But who can do this? Therefore, I am afraid that the farmer organizations and the mostly involved Federal States will be not very keen to enter the program. However, increasing import restrictions for pigs are to be expected in parallel to eradication of AD in some countries in the European Community. This will force the FRG to get free of AD. A precondition will be that the European Community gives financial support.

THE CONTROL PROGRAMME OF AUJESZKY'S DISEASE IN FRANCE: MAIN RESULTS AND DIFFICULTIES

P. Vannier

Ministère de l'Agriculture, D.G.A.L.
Station de Pathologie Porcine, BP 9, 22440 Ploufragan, France

ABSTRACT

Results obtained in different regions of France where medical or sanitary prohylaxises are applied to fight against Aujeszky's disease (AD) are compared. With sanitary measures, rapid and spectacular results have been obtained. The cost of these measures is dependent on the number of slaughtered animals; it was relatively low (US $ 4.8 per sow). In all the cases, medical measures are much more difficult to set up, to apply and to verify that the sanitary ones. Two different situations have to be considered. When a compulsory vaccination programme on breeders with serological tests on baconers has been decided, the degree of reliability of the measures and the results, after only a 1-year campaign, appear favourable at present. It is more difficult to evaluate the results in regions with a compulsory vaccination programme on breeding and fattening pigs. An epidemiological inquiry showed that classical vaccination schemes with 3 vaccines on fattening pigs do not seem to prevent or to limit the spread of wild-type virus in the herds. Under these conditions and in areas with a high density of pig herds, it can be assumed that virus transmission between animals and farms is still possible in spite of a generalized vaccination in fattening units. Consequently, in the case of epizootics of AD, where generalized medical prohylaxis is practised, the major property of the used vaccines should be the absence or very limited excretion of wild-type virus after infection of vaccinated pigs. The choice of using deleted vaccines is then of secondary importance. On the other hand, to eliminate latently infected breeders in herds where vaccination is practised, the use of deleted vaccines is fundamental. For that purpose, only glycoprotein I-negative inactivated virus vaccines are projected to be used on breeders in 2 French Departments in the short future.

INTRODUCTION

In France, there is several years of experience, with a control programme for Aujeszky's disease (AD) in most of the main producing regions, which at present comprise some 80% of the French pig production.

J. T. van Oirschot (ed.), Vaccination and Control of Aujeszky's Disease, 215–226.

Historical events

The history of AD in France can be divided into 3 periods: 1912-1967, 1968-1983, and 1984 until today. During the first period, clinical outbreaks of AD appeared sporadically: from 1912 to 1967, only 19 outbreaks have been recorded (Toma *et al.*, 1975). From 1968, each year the number of clinical outbreaks increased roughly (Toma *et al.*, 1975; Toma *et al.*, 1984). Furthermore, the number of administrative departments where AD outbreaks were observed for the first time regularly increased. Most of them have been recorded in Brittany: 210 outbreaks on a total of 344 in France in 1983 (61%) (Toma *et al.*, 1984). Consequently, numerous breeders were vaccinated in Brittany, particularly from 1975.

The years 1983-1984 were essential in the fight against AD. First, from 1983, the prevalence of AD among fattening units increased sharply. In Brittany, AD is no longer a major problem for piglets (due to the generalized vaccination of sows), but the virus persists and induces troubles in fattening units even if the breeders are vaccinated (Vannier, 1984). Second, on August 20, a national regulation was published defining the sanitary required conditions for the trade of breeding pigs. From 1984, measures were taken in different regions to control AD. The department of Loire-Atlantique was opening the way with a local regulation: compulsory registration of pig herds and exhaustive census, identification of all breeding herds, vaccination prohibited, except derogation, quarantaine and serological examination of bought breeders, annual serological survey of each herd, control of pig movements, definition of measures adopted in infected pig herds.

Epidemiological features

From the results of different epidemiological inquiries (Vannier, 1984; Baralon *et al.*, 1986; Darré *et al.*, 1986), which is supported by results of experimental infections (Donaldson *et al.,* 1983), 2 modes of spread of AD virus (ADV) seem to predominate in France. In Brittany, ADV multiplies actively in fattening pigs housed on industrial farms and seems mainly to be disseminated from farm to farm by airborne transmission. In other regions, infected breeders and particularly "traveling" boars are the main vectors of viral spread (Darré *et al.*, 1986). In that case, pigs and breeders raised in small size traditional farms are the main reservoirs of ADV.

FRENCH ERADICATION PROGRAMME AGAINST AUJESZKY'S DISEASE

The programme is based on the possibility to take various measures, dependable of the results of a preliminary serological survey, done on a representative sample of the pig population in the area concerned. Such a survey has to be done before any measure can be implemented. In addition, it is necessary to do an exhaustive census of the pig herds, to know exactly the distribution of farms and the number of pigs (Vannier and Le Foll, 1987). Fig. 1 shows that strict sanitary measures are implemented in the regions of Normandy, Pays de Loire, Poitou-Charentes, Aquitaine, Midi-Pyrénées and Languedoc. In these regions, vaccination is forbidden and a certain proportion of the breeding animals in each herd, related to the herd size, has to be examined each year. If infected pigs are detected,

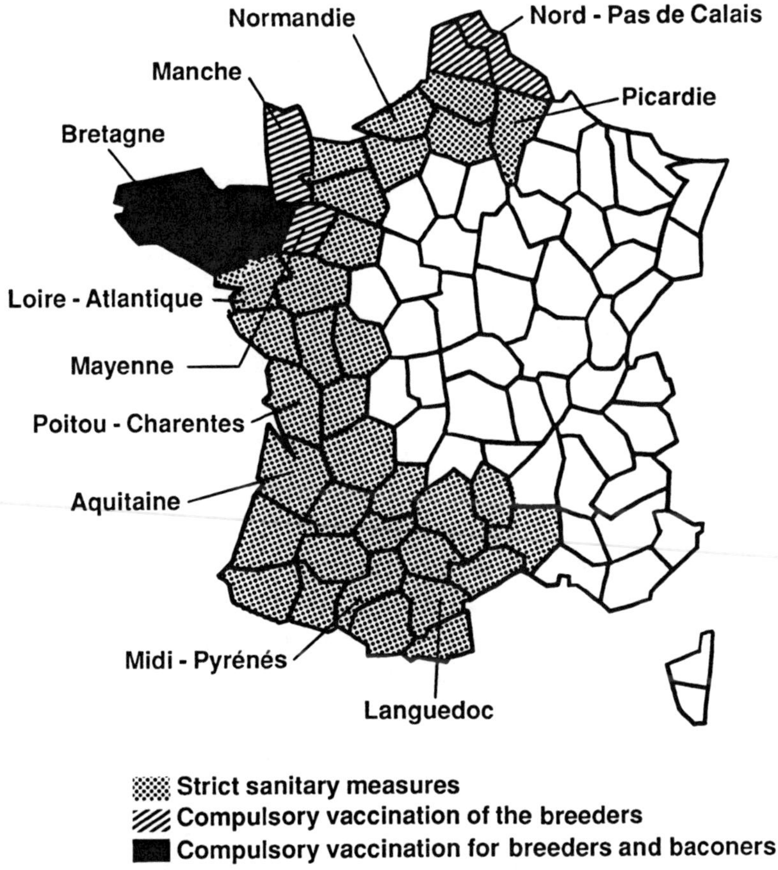

Fig. 1 Control programmes of Aujeszky's disease.

3 different measures can be decided; the decision being taken, case by case, by an official committee. These measures are: total or partial slaughter, or a special vaccination programme associated, after a certain time, with serological examinations on fattening pigs and breeders under the control of the veterinary services and for a limited time, according to the epidemiological risk for the neighbourhood. A financial compensation is given to the farmers which pay a levy. Local, regional and parapublic authorities also participate in the financing.

In other administrative departments, mainly to decrease the clinical risk, farmers decided to adopt a compulsory vaccination of the breeding pigs with a systematic serological screening of fattening pigs in each herd. These measures are always applied for a limited period and will be followed by strict sanitary measures. This has been done in areas of the departments of Nord, Pas de Calais, and Mayenne. In the 2 former departments, the exclusive use of glycoprotein I (gI) negative inactivated virus vaccines for breeders is projected to be imposed in a few months. Live virus vaccines are used, in a preventive way, in fattening pigs in certain areas of these departments. In these areas several cases of ADV infection were detected by the systemic serological survey done on fattening pigs.

For the other regions where prevalence of AD was higher, it was not possible to begin with a sanitary programme. So, a compulsory vaccination for breeding and fattening stock, with a strict administrative check of vaccination has been decided to be the first step in Brittany. Apart from these different measures, national rules determine the conditions of trade in breeding pigs from the 1100 selection and multiplication herds. All these herds have to be free of AD as evidenced by 4 yearly serological screenings of each herd.

RESULTS

Regions with a sanitary programme

Table 1 shows the results obtained after 1 or 2 campaigns. The measures taken were very effective, as the prevalence of infection decreased very quickly, even in departments where the original level of infection was high as in Pyrénées Atlantiques, Gers, Hautes-Pyrénées. A campaign is defined as the period required for the collection of blood samples, the analysis and application of measures decided in all the herd of the concerned area. Generally, a campaign lasts 1 year. The number of herds in Manche (Table 1) has to be considered an estimation, because it was not validated by the systemic serological check campaign of all the herds. Such a campaign allows to discover herds which have not previously been registered, and consequently refines the initial census. It has to be emphasized that, in Table 1, a herd is considered to be infected if only 1 pig is seropositive for AD. Usually, slaughter of only the infected animals sufficed to "clean up" the herd. In that case, the breeders were probably latently infected and virus was therefore not spread to other animals. However, partial slaughter have to be done rapidly to limit or avoid the risk of reactivation of ADV. The number of sows slaughtered in the last campaigns remained very low (Loire-Atlantique: 4, Vendée: 3, Landes: 1, Pyrénées Atlantiques: 42) (Vannier and Le Foll, 1988).

Generalized vaccination also appeared efficient in infected herds, provided they are applied rigourously and for at least 2 years. The department of Loire-Atlantique is probably the most experienced in this respect: In 1987, only 2 herds on a total of 245 had a derogation about vaccination. In the other herds, where the vaccination scheme was followed (2 in total), vaccination was stopped and the last vaccinated breeders present at the moment of infection were culled at a rate higher than the normal turn-over rate. Sera of breeders which were introduced later, and of baconers were free of antibodies against ADV.

In summary, the results obtained in numerous regions from one campaign to another are spectacular.

The cost of these measures can be evaluated in 2 regions. In Loire-Atlantique the programme began in 1983 and concerned a maximum of 247 herds. Over 3 years, the operation costed less than FF 900,000 (about US $ 145,000), including everything except the participation of the state veterinary services (blood sampling, laboratory analysis, vaccines, compensation, mortality, staff and travelling). As the programme has concerned 10,000 sows, the cost is FF 30 or US $4.8 per sow, per year. The levy paid by the farmers was FF 22 per sow, per year. The supplement came from the local or regional authorities and from the OFIVAL, which is a national parapublic organisation. The state veterinary services paid a part of the staff, and antigen for the serological tests (Vannier and Le Foll, 1988).

In the region of Aquitaine, where vaccination is now prohibited, after 2 years of prophylaxis 80,000 blood samples have been taken in 5,200 herds. From these samples, 3900 sows were infected and 4,200 have been slaughtered in the first stage of the eradication scheme. Here, the total cost has been 9 million francs (US $ 1.44 million) for 75,000 sows for 4 years, which is FF 30 per sow per year. The levy paid by the farmers for the first and second year was FF 10 per sow (=30%). In addition, 30% of the costs comes from OFIVAL and 25% from local authorities. The Ministry of Agriculture pays 5% and the regional authorities 10%. The levy paid by the farmers will increase slightly over the next 2 years.

TABLE 1 Results of sanitary measures adopted in different French regions. (Vannier and Le Foll, 1988)

REGIONS-DEPARTEMENTS	Total real number of breeding, breeding-fattening herds [1]	First campaign		Second campaign	
		Number of herds with blood samples	% of herds with infected animals	Number of herds with blood samples	% of herds with infected animals
PAYS DE LOIRE					
Loire-Atlantique	245	237	7,7	285	14,0
Maine-et-Loire	550	333	10,2		
Sarthe	576	401	2,2		
Vendée	233	227	2,6	230	0,4
ZONE AREPSA					
Dordogne	303	275	1,8		
Gironde	15	11	0	15	0
Landes	137	198	8,6	137	0,73
Lot-et-Garonne	114	141	7,1	114	0
Pyrénées-Atlantiques	1810	2100	18,0	1810	1,7
Ariège	32	41	2,4	32	0
Haute-Garonne	320	205	31,7		
Gers	382	494	15,2	382	1,3
Hautes-Pyrénées	1372	2115	23,3	1372	5,2
ZONE ASAMIP					
Aveyron	910	910	9,3		
Lot	236	236	4,7		
Tarn	276	276	4,0		
Tarn et Garonne	68	68	0		
NORMANDIE					
Eure	196	196	0,5	173	0
Seine-Maritime	170	145	0	121	0
Calvados	157	60	10 [2]	89	7,9 [2]
Manche	438 [3]	147	5,4	102	1,0
Orne	124	111	1,8	124	0

	Total real number of breeding, breeding-fattening herds (1)	Third campaign		Fourth campaign	
		Number of herds with blood samples	% of herds with infected animals	Number of herds with blood samples	% of herds with infected animals
Loire-Atlantique	245	248	2,4	245	1,2

[1] Number obtained from the last census done at the moment of the most recent campaign
[2] Vaccinated animals included
[3] The last campaign indicated has been done between 1986-1987. The previous ones correspond to the previous 12 months period.

Regions with a medical programme

It is too early to deal with results but epidemiological features are interesting. It is necessary to distinguish between the departments of Nord and Pas de Calais, where AD outbreaks occur sporadically, and Brittany where AD is widespread.

In the departments of Nord and Pas de Calais the situation appears favourable. The percentages of vaccinated breeders, and examined and infected herds are given in Table 2. In medical areas only the breeders are vaccinated. Serological examination is done on baconers in farrow-to-finishing herds.

TABLE 2 Situation in Nord and Pas-de-Calais departments

Department	Medical area	Sanitary area
Nord	77% breeders vaccinated Blood samples on baconers in 74% of farrow-to-finishing herds	Blood samples on breeders in 75% herds
	Infection rate 28/436 herds: 6.4%	Infection rate 24/372: 6.4%
Pas de Calais	80% breeders vaccinated in 746/1280 (58%) herds Blood samples on baconers in 70% of farrow-to-finishing herds	Blood samples on breeders in 50 to 90% of herds
	4 infected herds in 1987	

A systemic preventive vaccination of fattening pigs is applied in the Nord department, only in small areas with a high rate of infection, which corresponds often with a higher density of pig farms. Vaccination is not justified in the other parts of the Nord department. In medical areas, vaccination of breeders with gI-negative inactivated virus vaccines will be soon applied to begin eradication of AD under a vaccinal protection.

In Brittany, it is presently not possible to evaluate the degree of reliability of the measures in the whole region. An epidemiological inquiry has been done in an area with a high density of pig farms, where a compulsory vaccination programme on both breeders and baconers is applied. Actually, 3 vaccines (A, B and C) are used in fattening pigs. In this survey, 10 blood samples of baconers per herd have been collected at the end of the fattening period. Samples have been collected on 128 vaccinated fattening units from breeding and finishing herds.

Figs. 2, 3 and 4 show the distribution of the sera of pigs vaccinated with either of the 3 vaccines according to their virus neutralizing (VN) antibody titres, measured in a 1-hour neutralization test. They indicate a wide variability of individual antibody responses after vaccination. This variability results from differences in the administration of the vaccines and from differences in the level of passive immunity at the moment of vaccination. From experimental data obtained by vaccination of pigs with each of the 3 vaccines, followed by challenge at the end of the fattening period, it seems possible to define a serological profile of vaccinated and infected pigs. By using a standardized neutralization test, it is, therefore, possible to detect,

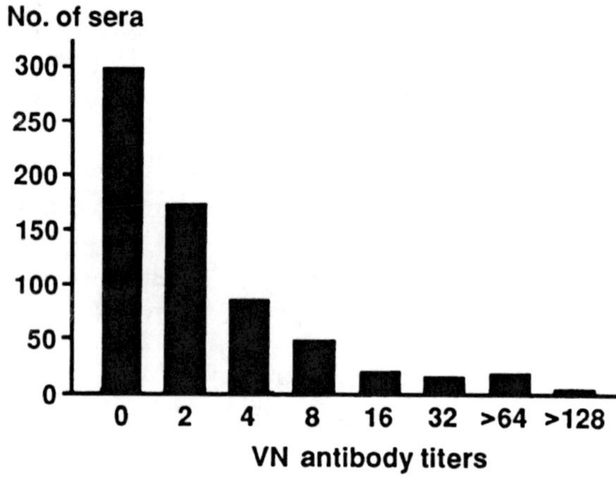

Fig. 2 Distribution of sera of pigs vaccinated with vaccine A according to their VN antibody titers.

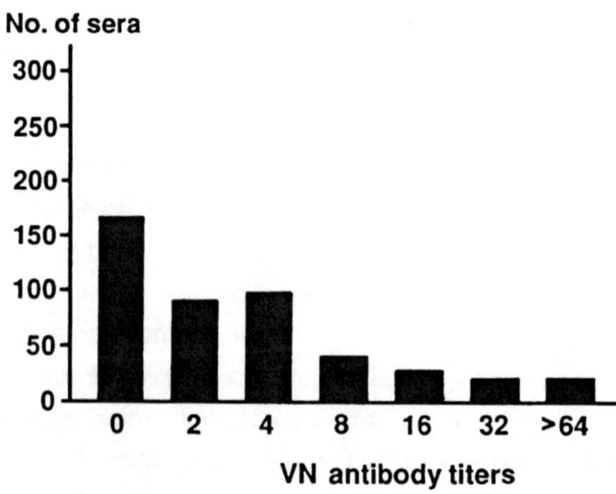

Fig. 3 Distribution of sera of pigs vaccinated with vaccine B according to their VN antibody titers.

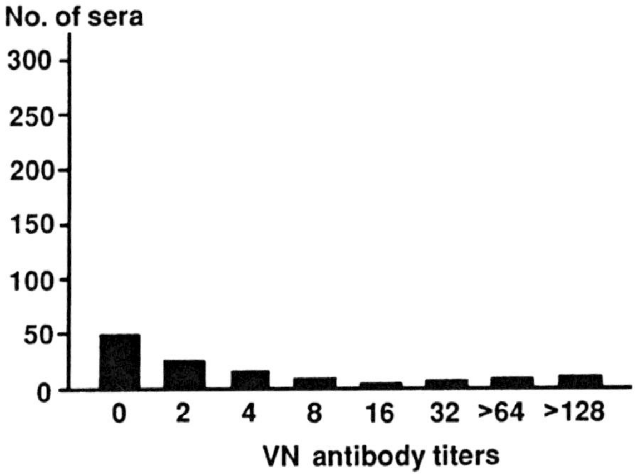

Fig. 4 Distribution of sera of pigs vaccinated with vaccine C according to their VN antibody titers.

with a small chance of error, a recent infection in a vaccinated herd. High VN antibody titres found in sera of fattening pigs just before slaughter is in all probability due to an ADV infection. Using the above criterion, 23 of the 128 vaccinated breeder-fattening herds can considered to be infected. This approach has been validated in 45 herds, where pigs were vaccinated with the gI-negative vaccine B (Eloit *et al.*, 1988). Table 3 shows that in these 45 herds 4 were considered to be infected from data obtained by analyzing the VN antibody titres, whereas 6 were considered as infected by using the ELISA technique to differentiate antibodies induced by vaccination or infection (Eloit *et al.*, 1988).

Table 3 Number of herds considered to be infected with ADV.

Method used	Number of herds Considered as infected	Doubtful results	Total
Neutralisation test	4	2	45
Differentiation ELISA test	6	4	

From the sera collected in the infected herds 64% may be considered as sampled from an infected pig. These data demonstrate that the adopted compulsory vaccination programme does not seem to prevent dissemination of ADV in and perhaps among pig herds. But additional data are needed to confirm these preliminary results.

DISCUSSION

Sanitary measures were always successful in the control of AD in France. The chosen strategy has to be adapted to the local epidemiological situation. At midterm, the cost of these measures were relatively low.

Medical measures were much more difficult to set up, to apply and to verify than the sanitary ones. Moreover, because farmers themselves vaccinate their pigs, there are qualitative differences in the administration of vaccines. Vaccination schemes of fattening pigs, as indicated by the manufacturers, may not uniformly prevent or, sometimes, even limit the spread of field virus in herds. Therefore, virus transmission between pigs and perhaps airborne transmission of ADV between farms may still be possible in spite of generalized vaccination of fattening units. Thus, the question arises, whether eradication of AD is possible with a generalized vaccination campaign in areas with a high density of pig farms and a high prevalence of ADV infection. Anyway, it appears to be clear, that, in a setting of a medical prophylaxy, the control strategy should be different when the infection runs an epizootic course, particularly in fatteners, or when the infections are mainly latent in breeders. In the former case, the choice of an appropriate vaccination scheme of fattening pigs is the major point in the decided strategy. The chosen vaccines have to limit or even discontinue the viral excretion after infection of pigs. With regard to eradication this vaccinal property is of higher importance than the clinical protection. But, there is no data available about the comparison of different vaccines on the viral excretion after infection of vaccinated animals. Moreover, it would be difficult to extrapolate experimental results obtained with a limited numer of animals with the high "infectious pressure" observed in fattening units housing several hundreds of animals. In this context, the choice for deleted virus vaccines is of secondary importance, because knowledge of the presence of virus in fattening units is not really useful, since the risk of long or short distance transmission of virus is always present before the detection of infection by serological tests. Thus from an epidemiological, as well as from an economical, point of view slaughtering of infected fatteners is totally unjustified. On the other hand, tracing of ADV infected fattening herds is interesting, because it reveals precisely the real epidemiological situation in an area.

In breeding herds the association of medical prophylaxis and accelarated culling of sows can lead to elimination of latently infected animals from a herd (McCracken *et al.*, 1984; Vannier *et al.*, 1984). The use of deleted virus vaccines is in this case fundamental and is the only way to set up such sanitary measures with a clinical passive protection of pigs induced by the systemic vaccination of the dams. However, with regard to the epidemiological situation in the different regions of France, it can be assumed that this prophylactic stage is a final one. The size of the sampling of the breeding population has to be determined as systemic vaccination probably modifies the course of an ADV infection. It does not seem to be realistic to collect serum of every breeder in a farm in the setting of a permanent eradication programme, e.g., which has to be done at least once a year in each herd. In that sense, the future experiences in Nord and Pas de Calais, where only gI-negative inactivated virus vaccines will be used for breeding pigs, while the fatteners remain unvaccinated, will be interesting to follow.

All these observations demonstrate the vital importance of cooperation between the different European countries. This cooperation is particulary important for the trade of breeding animals (which have to be free of ADV antibodies) when control measures are harmonized, and for the protection of countries considered free of AD. For example, it becomes possible to plan a compulsory generalized vaccination for certain regions of West Germany, close to the Danish border, where ADV is prevalent, to offer a better protection for the AD free herds in Denmark. The absence of prophylaxis in Belgium creates real problems in the 2 French Departments on the other side of the border. At term, such a situation could annihilate efforts done in France. Such harmonized actions could be of greater value, when the importance of the airborne transmission of ADV is better understood.

ACKNOWLEDGEMENTS

The author wishes to thank Dr. Gouëllo and his team, M. Colcanap, Botrel, Briand, Le Picard (D.D.S.V., Place du 71e RI, St Brieuc 22000), who participated to the epidemiological inquiry in the setting of medical prophylaxy. I thank P. Le Foll (ITP, Le Rheu 35650), who collected with me the data in regions with a sanitary program. I thank all the people responsible for the regional coordination of eradication programs against AD, the Unions Régionales des Groupements de Producteurs de Porcs, the Fédérations Régionales de Groupements de Défense Sanitaire du Bétail, the Directions Départementales des Services Vétérinaires, the Fédérations Départementales de Groupement de Défense Sanitaire du Bétail for their help to collect the presented data. I want to thank also J.P. Delalande for his helpful technical assistance.

REFERENCES

Baralon, P., Berges, M., Chantal, J., Daridan, D., Darré, R. and Le Foll, P. 1986. Réalisation d'une enquête épidémiologique concernant la maladie d'Aujeszky dans le Sud-Ouest de la France. Note 1: Protocole de l' enquête. Rev. Med. Vet., **137,** 263-271.

Darré, R., Baralon, P., Berges, M., Chantal, J., Daridan, D. and Le Foll, P. 1986. Réalisation d'une enquête épidémiologique concernant la maladie d'Aujeszky dans le Sud-Ouest de la France. Note 2: Résultats et discussion. Rev. Med. Vet., **137,** 367-375.

Donaldson, A.I., Wardley, R.E., Martin, S. and Ferries, N.P. 1983. Experimental Aujeszky's disease in pigs: excretion, survival and transmission of the virus. Vet. Rec., **113,** 490-494.

Eloit, M., Fargeaud, D., Vannier, P. and Toma, B. 1988. Differentiation between pigs infected by Aujeszky's disease virus and pigs vaccinated with gI-negative strains. In: CEC Seminar on "Vaccination and control of Aujeszky's disease" (Ed. J.T. van Oirschot). (Kluwer Academic Publishers, Dordrecht).

McCracken, R.M., McFerran, J.B., McParland, P.J. and McKillop, E.R. 1984. Vaccination against Aujeszky's disease: field experience. Proc. 8th IPVS Congress, p. 35.

Toma, B., Le Turdu, Y. and Goret, P. 1975. Epidémiologie de la maladie d'Aujeszky en France. Bull. Off. Int. Epiz., **201,** 1-14.

Toma, B., Lorant, J.M., Vigouroux, A., Ursache, R., Bijlenga, G., David, C., Eloit, M., Duée, J.P., Rose, R., Alamagny, A., Le Gardinier, J.C. and Laurent, J. 1984. La maladie d'Aujeszky en France. Rec. Med. Vet. **160,** 563-568.

Vannier, P., Chermat, M., Bourgoin, J.C. and Simmoneau, M. 1984. Attempts to control and eliminate the Aujeszky's disease infection from 2 herds of swine by vaccination with an inactivated virus vaccine. Proc. 8th IPVS Congress, p. 44.

Vannier, P. 1984. La maladie d'Aujeszky: résultats d'une enquête épidémiologique en Bretagne. Bull. Lab. Vet., **13,** 1-11.

Vannier, P. and Le Foll, P. 1987. Comparing actions against Aujeszky's disease in Europe. Pig Int., **3,** 18-24.

Vannier, P. and Le Foll, P. 1988. Les grandes maladies virales contagieuses du porc: situation épidémiologique en France et en Europe. J. Rech. Porc., **20,** 73-82.

CONTROL OF AUJESZKY'S DISEASE IN GREECE. THE VIEW FROM A COUNTRY THAT IMPORTS A GREAT PART OF ITS SWINE BREEDING STOCK

O. Papadopoulos

Department of Infectious Diseases, School of Veterinary Medicine
Aristotelian University, 54006 Thessaloniki, Greece

ABSTRACT

A cluster of serious outbreaks was recorded in large farms following the introduction of imported breeding stock in 1983. Since then, imported pigs are serologically tested on a voluntary basis, and the number of positives has been reduced. Only killed vaccines have been licenced. The protection of Aujeszky's disease free farms is important, but the variety of control approaches in the exporting countries is an obstacle. Therefore, an acceptable common policy is necessary.

INTRODUCTION

Aujeszky's disease (AD) in Greece was first reported in cattle in 1952 and later in sheep, goats and mink; these cases were directly or indirectly connected with swine (Papadopoulos, 1974). Clinical disease in swine was reported much later (Stoforos, 1977) and followed the development of the intensive pig industry in the 1970's.

In 1978 AD was declared notifiable. New reported outbreaks were 0 in 1979, 1 in 1980, 0 in 1981, 3 in 1982, 20 in 1983, 2 in 1984, 6 in 1985, 6 in 1986 and 5 in 1987.

CONTROL MEASURES

The cluster of 20 outbreaks in 1983 shocked the pig industry. The most important cases occurred in large farms, shortly after the introduction of imported breeding stock. Control measures included temporary isolation of the infected farm and vaccination. Only killed vaccines have been licenced.

Following the outbreaks of 1983, almost all imported pigs were tested on arrival by virus neutralization test, on a voluntary basis, on the application of the importer.

J. T. van Oirschot (ed.), Vaccination and Control of Aujeszky's Disease, 227–229.

In case of positive reactions (a titer of 1:2 or higher), which meant infection or vaccination, the matter was settled between importer and exporter, according to their private agreement. For pigs imported from non-EEC countries, freedom from AD was mandatory.

The results of tests made by one diagnostic laboratory (State Veterinary Institute, Thessaloniki, Northern Greece) have been reported (Paschaleri *et al.*, 1987) and are shown in Table 1.

Positive reactions were reported as infection, because differentiation between infection and vaccination was not possible, at that time. A reduction of the number of positives is evident. It is believed to be the result of the awareness of the importing farmers, who preferred exporters that could provide seronegative animals.

TABLE 1 Serological tests for AD antibody in imported pigs (Paschaleri et al., 1987).

Origin	1983	1984	1985	1986	1987
Belgium	32:199*	—	—	—	—
Denmark	3: 30	4:147	0: 42	3:258	0: 38
Germany (FRG)	—	41: 93	0: 20	0: 39	—
Italy	—	104:113	—	—	—
The Netherlands	—	45:168	—	21:169	—
United Kingdom	6: 99	0:225	0:714	0:609	0:149
Austria	—	0: 20	0: 28	0: 19	—
Hungary	—	—	—	—	0: 15
Sweden	0: 36	—	—	0: 38	0: 40
Yugoslavia	—	—	—	0:104	—
Total	41:364	194:766	0:804	24:1136	0:242
%	(11%)	(25%)	(0)	(2%)	(0)

* = Positive: Tested

CONCLUSIONS

A state or industry controlled eradication program for AD is not applied in Greece. Awareness and technical assistance to farmers, when they buy breeding stock is an alternative. Protection of industrial farms that are not infected is of paramount importance. These are the farms that usually import their breeding stock. The variety of control strategies applied in the exporting countries is an obstacle, complicating control after arrival. Therefore, an acceptable common policy is desirable. Different, but compatible strategies may be a first step towards that purpose.

REFERENCES

Papadopoulos, O. 1974. La maladie d'Aujeszky en Grece. Cah. Med. Vet., **43,** 237-239.

Paschaleri, E., Papakostaki, D. and Kakamoukas, K. 1987. Aujeszky's disease in Northern Greece. Bull. Hell. Vet. Med. Ass., **40**, (in press).

Stoforos, E., Mastroyianni, M., Axiotis, I., Hatzimanolakis, K., Anagnostou, L., Loupis, S. and Loukas, S. 1977. Isolation of Aujeszky's disease virus from piglets. Bull. Hell. Vet. Med. Soc., **28,** 89.

VACCINATION AND CONTROL OF AUJESZKY'S DISEASE IN NORTHERN IRELAND

S.J. McCullough

Veterinary Research Laboratories
Stormont
Belfast, BT4 3SD
Northern Ireland

ABSTRACT

Aujeszky's disease virus infection is widespread in Northern Ireland pig herds. Vaccination has been used as a method of control since 1972. Eradication of infection is encouraged in pedigree breeding herds and vaccine has been of use in eliminating infection on some farms. Recent work on the epidemiology of the disease has led to a fuller understanding of some previously anomalous field observations. Developments in vaccine technology and in serology present new opportunities for achievement of countrywide eradication as a long term objective.

INTRODUCTION

Aujeszky's disease (AD) has long been recognised in pig herds in Northern Ireland (Lamont and Shanks, 1939). Infection is widespread, with antibody present in 50% of herds of 50 or more breeding sows and 18% of fattening herds as determined by a survey carried out in 1978 (McCracken *et al.*, 1984). Though the disease is not of major economic concern to the industry as a whole, it is important to those producers who suffer loss directly through clinical disease or indirectly through inability to sell valuable breeding stock because they carry antibody and by implication are potentially a source of infection.

Outbreaks tend to be sporadic in occurrence and were generally self-limiting in small herds before vaccines were used. In other countries, the disease became more important to some producers in the early 1970's as the structure of the pig industry changed towards a smaller number of larger units where infection could become endemic (Cartwright, 1982; Lenihan and O'Connor, 1982). At about the same time, the emergence of highly virulent strains of Aujeszky's disease virus (ADV) was an additional complication in the control of the disease in Northern Ireland.

In 1972 vaccine was first used to control an outbreak of disease on a large

J. T. van Oirschot (ed.), Vaccination and Control of Aujeszky's Disease, 231–238.

fattening unit where the clinical signs were particularly severe and mortality rates were up to 13% in 12 to 16-week-old pigs. A live vaccine containing the Bartha strain of ADV was prepared at Stormont and successfully controlled the outbreak (McFerran and Dow, 1975). In subsequent outbreaks on the same site, vaccination was successfully carried out using the NIA-4 strain (McFerran *et al.*, 1982).

Further severe outbreaks in other herds led to a policy decision that vaccine should be available for the control of disease in commercial units, though eradication should be encouraged in pedigree breeding herds. This policy remains unchanged at present.

THE EPIDEMIOLOGY OF ADV

Recent work at Stormont has been aimed at a fuller understanding of the epidemiology of AD including observations on the spread of infection in some herds which could not be explained in terms of the characteristics of the known strains of ADV. A more complete understanding of the epidemiology of the disease will allow informed decisions to be made on any future eradication scheme.

Subclinical infection

Outbreaks of clinical disease have been diagnosed at a rate of 20-30 per year. This has been fairly constant over the years despite the use of vaccines. McFerran and Dow (1965) first suggested that much of the infection must be subclinical since antibody is so widespread. Some infection with virulent strains probably takes place in non-pregnant older pigs, resulting in insignificant clinical signs. However, the possibility of subclinical infection of susceptible young pigs with low doses of virulent virus has not been investigated. A low infection dose may result in a low level of virus excretion and hence the spread of subclinical infection.

Experimental infection of groups of 4-week-old pigs with different doses of the NIA-2 strain of ADV indicated a minimum infectious dose of approximately 100 50% tissue culture infectious doses ($TCID_{50}$). The groups of pigs inoculated with 100 and 1000 TCID50 developed clinical signs as severe as those in groups of pigs given higher doses, though seroconversion, virus excretion and the development of clinical signs were delayed for a period inversely related to the dose. The low doses of virus were probably multiplied by cross-infection within the groups of pigs during this period, so it is unlikely that virulent strains such as NIA-2 could cause subclinical infection of young susceptible pigs under field conditions.

Spreading subclinical infection was monitored on 1 farm and a new strain of

ADV (NIA-6) was isolated as a result (McCullough and Todd, 1988). Experimental infections using this strain have shown that it is avirulent in 4-week-old pigs, yet infection is naturally transmissible which differentiates it from the avirulent bovine isolate NIA-4. Spread of NIA-6 within the animal was slow, limited in extent and quickly cleared when compared to that following experimental infection with the virulent NIA-1 strain.

The spread of infection on the original farm was slow and no clinical signs were seen though seroconversion was detected in very young piglets. However, experimental intranasal inoculation of high doses of NIA-6 resulted in severe clinical signs and high mortality in 2-week-old pigs. Fatally infected pigs transmitted infection to in-contacts but no clinical signs were recorded in the latter, so the doses of virus given experimentally ($10^{5.8}$ and $10^{7.5}$ $TCID_{50}$) were probably higher than those encountered in natural infection and in infection by contact. ADV strains similar to NIA-6 could account for subclinical infection in the field.

Serological results from other herds have established that it is not uncommon that there is a small number of seropositive animals in a herd and no clinical disease. Transmission of infection seems to be limited and, in some herds where new stock have been tested and quarantined to prevent the introduction of a more virulent strain, infection had spontaneously died out. Since NIA-6 infection has been shown to spread, albeit slowly, there may be field strains of even lower virulence. The extent of subclinical infection in Northern Ireland herds is not known but available evidence suggests that it is widespread.

Virus virulence and the spread of infection

Field isolates of ADV in Northern Ireland have been shown to vary in virulence and in tissue tropism (Table 1) (Dow and McFerran, 1962; McFerran and Dow, 1965; Baskerville *et al.*, 1973; McFerran and Dow, 1975; McCullough and Todd, 1988). The recent isolation of the NIA-6 strain has extended the range of virulence of the

TABLE 1 The virulence and tissue tropism of Northern Ireland isolates of ADV

Strain	Species of origin	Virulence in pigs 2 wks	4 wks	8 wks	12 wks	Tissue tropism CNS	Lung
NIA-1	Pig	+ + + +	+ + + +	+ +	—	+	—
NIA-2	Pig	+ + + +	+ + + +	+ +	—	+	+ +
NIA-3	Pig	+ + + +	+ + + +	+ + + +	+ + + +	+	+/—
NIA-4	Cattle	—	—	—	—	+	—
NIA-6	Pig	+ +	—	—	—	+	—

field isolates from pigs. Field observations and the results of experimental work have indicated that there is a relationship between virulence and ability to spread.

The infectious dose of NIA-6 may be higher than that of a more virulent strain or it may be that less virus is excreted as a result of infection; both these factors may be important. A series of experiments were carried out to determine the ID_{50} for each of the 3 field strains NIA-2, -3 and -6. Each pig was kept in isolation to avoid cross-infection and 4 pigs were intranasally (IN) inoculated at each dose level. The results are shown in Table 2. It is clear that the ID_{50} is inversely proportional to virulence. Virus excretion is difficult to quantify, but the virus content of tonsil swabs taken from the above pigs was compared and it was found that less virus was detected in swabs taken from pigs infected with NIA-6 than from those infected with NIA-2; these pigs were IN inoculated with a dose 10 times greater than the respective ID_{50}.

TABLE 2 Virulence and the infectious dose of Northern Ireland isolated of ADV

Strain	Virulence	ID_{50}/Log10 $TCID_{50}$
NIA-3	High	1.5
NIA-2	Medium	2.5
NIA-6	Low	5.0

Thus the more virulent the strain of ADV, the more readily it will spread. In much of the work on the efficacy of vaccines, highly virulent strains have been used as challenge virus and, while it has been shown that vaccination does not prevent infection with or excretion of challenge virus in these circumstances (McFerran *et al.*, 1982; Donaldson *et al.*, 1984; De Leeuw and Van Oirschot, 1985), it may be more effective against less virulent strains. However, virus excretion is reduced in vaccinated pigs and field experience has shown that vaccination does reduce spread, even when the strain of virus is highly virulent.

VACCINATION AND CONTROL OF AD

The present situation

An attenuated live vaccine based on the Bartha K61 strain of ADV is presently used in Northern Ireland, though generally only in response to outbreaks of clinical disease. The other aspect of control is the encouragement of pedigree breeding herds to eradicate infection. A register of ADV free herds has been set up to facilitate the sale of breeding stock and the movement of animals to shows, sales and to the performance testing centre. Two antibody free herd tests at an interval of at least 4 months are required to qualify for the register and screening tests are carried out at 6 monthly intervals thereafter. Owners are recommended to buy only serologically negative animals, to quarantine them on the farm for 2 weeks and then to retest before moving seronegative pigs into the herd.

Several methods have been applied in the eradication of infection on a herd basis:

1. De-stocking the infected premises, disinfection and restocking with uninfected pigs. This method is the most expensive and is not applicable where the herd consists of valuable breeding lines which the owner wishes to conserve.
2. A nucleus herd made up of antibody-free animals can be moved to an uninfected accommodation separated from the original farm which is then gradually destocked while the numbers of pigs in the nucleus herd is built up. The nucleus herd must be carefully isolated and the pigs regularly monitored for seroconversion to ADV. The pigs in the original herd may be vaccinated to reduce the amount of virus excretion and when the infected pigs have been cleared out, the houses are disinfected before the nucleus herd is moved back. By this method, valuable breeding lines can be conserved if sufficient numbers of suitable, uninfected pigs are available. Access to appropriate housing for the nucleus herd and the difficulties in avoiding cross-infection are 2 of the limiting factors.
3. In herds where there are only a small number of seropositive pigs, a programme of serological testing and culling of seropositive pigs has been successful. Several cycles of testing and culling may be required. Where the low percentage infection in a herd can be shown to have been static over a period of years, this implies that a strain of ADV of low virulence may be responsible. If so, the spread of infection will be slow and this method is the more likely to be successful. Particularly in small units, a past outbreak of the disease involving a more virulent strain may have been selflimiting and the small number of seropositive pigs would then represent the survivors and they could be a source of latent virulent virus which could make eradication more difficult.
4. McCracken *et al.* (1984) showed that vaccination of all pigs in a herd for a long period of time may eradicate field virus infection. Vaccination reduces the amount of circulating virus and no new infections occur so that eventually, as older pigs are culled, all the remainder have antibody induced by vaccine and none are latently infected. At this point, vaccination is stopped and the young, unvaccinated pigs are

used as sentinels for field virus. If they remain free of clinical signs and antibody, eradication has been achieved; if not, vaccination must be restarted and the process repeated. If this method of eradication is successful, the herd cannot join the register of ADV free herds until all the vaccinated animals have been culled. In herds where this method has not been successful it is likely that the recommended hygienic measures have not been followed and a new field strain of ADV has been introduced during the vaccination period. The new infection is impossible to trace and results in the reappearance of field virus once vaccination is stopped.

The most common method of transmission of infection from one herd to another is by the transfer of infected animals so the test and quarantine procedure for the introduction of new stock is vitally important and, where 1 of the above methods of eradication has failed it is often because this has not been done.

The ADV ELISA described by Todd *et al.*(1981) is used in serological testing and the adaptation of this test for filter paper discs (Banks, 1985) has been readily adopted for the testing of large numbers of pigs.

Future prospects

The use of vaccine over a number of years has not reduced the number or severity of outbreaks of AD and, although it has helped in eradication on a herd basis, infection is still widespread. The sporadic nature of the use of vaccine in outbreaks of clinical disease has been ineffective in reducing the circulation of field virus strains. Countrywide eradication is a desirable long-term objective but the methods available to achieve it are limited. Testing and slaughter of all seropositive animals as in England and Wales is not practicable because infection is so widespread and because of the use of vaccine. Any eradication scheme is likely to have to be financed by the industry, so must be economically attractive.

The benefits of eradication in terms of avoidance of direct losses due to clinical disease are likely to be small in relation to the cost of controlling a disease with such a high prevalence of infection. The maintenance of markets for pigs and pigmeat products will be the most significant economic factor influencing the decision on eradication.

Recent developments in vaccine technology and in serology have resulted in several methods of differentiating vaccinated animals from those infected with field strains of ADV and these present new possibilities for the control or eradication of the disease.

1. A more efficient method of eradication by vaccination since infection with field strains could be monitored independently, allowing the decision on when to stop

vaccinating to be made with confidence.

2. The introduction of infection into a vaccinated herd could be detected.

3. Pigs seropositive to field strains of ADV could be identified and culled while the rest of the herd is protected by vaccination.

4. Vaccine could be used in herds where ADV has been eradicated if there was a risk of reinfection.

5. Eradication of AD in Northern Ireland by vaccination could become cost-effective. Losses through clinical disease could be eliminated without jeopardising export markets.

However, the economic benefits of the opportunities for control of AD presented by the new technology depend largely upon harmonisation of approach within the European Community. In the case of Northern Ireland, it is particularly important that we adopt a policy which is compatible with that in the Republic of Ireland.

REFERENCES

Banks, M. 1985. Detection of antibodies to Aujeszky's disease virus in whole blood by Elisadisc. J. Virol. Meth., **12**, 41-45.

Baskerville, A., McFerran, J.B. and Dow, C. 1973. Aujeszky's disease in pigs. Vet. Bull., **43**, 465-480.

Cartwright, S. 1982. Epidemiology and control of Aujeszky's disease in Great Britain. Ref.: Curr. Top. Vet. Med. Am. Sci., **17**,237-244. In: CEC Seminar on "Aujeszky's Disease" (Eds. G.A. Wittmann and S.A. Hall). (Martinus Nijhoff, The Hague).

Donaldson, A.I., Wardley, R.C., Martin, S., Harkness, J.W. 1984. Influence of vaccination on Aujeszky's disease virus and disease transmission. Vet. Rec., **115**, 121-124.

De Leeuw, P.W. and Van Oirschot, J.T. 1985. Vaccines against Aujeszky's disease; evaluation of their efficacy under standardised laboratory conditions. Vet. Quart., **7**, 191-197.

Dow, C. and McFerran, J.B. 1962. The neuropathology of Aujeszky's disease in the pig. Res. Vet. Sci., **3**, 436-442.

Lamont, H.G. and Shanks, P.L. 1939. An outbreak of Aujeszky's disease amongst pigs. Vet. Rec., **51**, 1407-1408.

Lenihan, P. and O'Connor, P.J. 1982. Epidemiology and control of Aujeszky's disease in the Republic of Ireland. Ref.: Curr. Top. Vet. Med. Am. Sci., **17**, 157-162. In: CEC Seminar on "Aujeszky's disease" (Eds. G. Wittmann and S.A. Hall). (Martinus Nijhoff, The Hague).

McCracken, R.M., McFerran, J.B., McParland, P.J. and McKillop, E.R. 1984. Vaccination against Aujeszky's disease: Field experiences. Vet. Rec., **115**, 348-352.

McCullough, S.J. and Todd, D. 1988. Subclinical Aujeszky's disease virus infection in a pig herd and the characterisation of the strain of virus isolated. Vet. Rec., **122**, 77-81.

McFerran, J.B.and Dow, C. 1965. The distribution of the virus of Aujeszky's disease (pseudorabies) in experimentally infected swine. Am. J. Vet. Res., **26**, 631-635.

McFerran, J.B. and Dow, C. 1975. Studies on immunisation of pigs with the Bartha strain of Aujeszky's disease virus. Res. Vet. Sci., **19**, 17-22.

McFerran, J.B., McCracken, R.M. and Dow, C. 1982. Comparative studies with inactivated and attenuated vaccines for protection of fattening pigs. Ref.: Curr. Top. Vet. Med. Am. Sci., **17**, 163-170. In: CEC Seminar on "Aujeszky's disease" (Eds. G. Wittmann and S.A. Hall). (Martinus Nijhoff, The Hague).

Todd, D., McNair, J., McNulty, M.S. and McFerran, J.B. 1981. Enzyme linked immunosorbent assay for detecting antibodies to Aujeszky's disease virus in pigs. Vet. Rec., **109**, 534-537.

ERADICATION AND CONTROL OF AUJESZKY'S DISEASE IN THE GERMAN DEMOCRATIC REPUBLIC

Ch. Kretzschmar

Bezirkinstitut für Veterinärwesen
3500 Stendal, German Democratic Republic

ABSTRACT

In the strive for eradication of Aujeszky's disease (AD) it should be recognized that there are essential and nonessential measures, which are dependent on some important epizootiological factors.

Essential measures are:

1. Regular serological control of all swine herds, because in a considerable number of herds the infection runs a subclinical course.

2. All infected herds where a clinical, virological or serological diagnosis is made must be excluded from swine trade, because trade is the most important factor favouring spread of AD.

3. Vaccination should only "metaphylactically" be practised in infected herds and not in free herds. Consequently, each serological reaction in a free herd signalizes an infection with field virus.

4. Vaccinated herds must be excluded from swine trade, because latency of field virus is not abolished by vaccination and because vaccination, moreover, does not absolutely prevent infection and subsequent latency of field virus.

5. Vaccination should be practised in as many infected herds as possible for reducing virus multiplication and consequently the spread of the infection.

6. Complete replacement of infected herds by stamping-out or fattening of those herds under the cover of vaccination is the best method for eradicating the infection. However, if the contact between infected and uninfected animals can be discontinued by stopping internal pig movements and the addition of pigs to the herd, one can succeed, even in large herds, in eliminating the field virus by a transient strict vaccination programme, until the breeding or fattening pigs have completely been replaced.

With the above strategical concept on the basis of stately ordered eradication programme and economic regulations for herd owners AD was eradicated in the German Democratic Republic in 1985. The 5 isolated cases that occurred since that time were related to neighbouring countries where the infection is enzootic. The yearly serological survey of all swine herds is to be continued.

INTRODUCTION

In 1985 eradication of Aujeszky's disease (AD) has been accomplished in the German Democratic Republic. A national uniform control programme based on new

J. T. van Oirschot (ed.), Vaccination and Control of Aujeszky's Disease, 239–247.

government regulations was implemented in 1966. The programme continually improved and new, more specific, legislation was introduced in 1976. Since that time several unexpected findings were made, especially in relation with the increase and intensifying of pig production in the sixties and the seventies. Finally in 1981, these developments lead to the decision to follow a stamping-out policy for the remaining infected herds. The national insurance on infectious animal diseases virtually financed the entire stamping-out programme.

Already for a long time, the existing scientific knowledge on AD sufficed to eradicate the disease and its causative virus. However, to achieve this goal, a tight organisation and continual control under primary responsibility of the Veterinary Service, based on legislative measures, were required. With regard to an eradication strategy for AD, it is essential to take into account some specific factors of epizootiological importance. If just one of these determining factors is overlooked, eradication of AD will not be accomplished. This paper largely deals with these determining factors and their consequences for the eradication of AD.

EPIZOOTIOLOGICAL FEATURES AND CONSEQUENCES FOR ERADICATION

First determining factor

Infections with AD virus (ADV) is neither in every pig nor in every pig herd associated with the appearance of clear clinical signs. Suckling piglets are often severely affected, but in fattening herds the infection is often not recognized. Even in larger breeding herds loss of suckling piglets may not occur, when ADV is primarily restricted to the buildings where sows without piglets are housed. These sows produce antibodies to protect their next litter.

Consequence

All breeding pig herds that in some way or another are involved in pig trade, must undergo a regular serological screening. At regular time intervals, randomly collected blood samples of closed herds and fattening herds must be serologically tested in order to identify subclinically infected herds. Since 1969, a yearly serological survey have been performed on all pig premises.

At the most intensive period during the eradication scheme, 700,000 to 1,000,000 samples were yearly examined in all regional animal health institutes. For this purpose, a standardized neutralization test was used.

Second determining factor

Once a pig has been infected and recovered it must be regarded as a lifelong potential source of virus spread. Most pigs that recover from AD are latently infected, and due to hardly defined circumstances virus reactivation and subsequent exretion may be induced, which may lead to recrudescent infections in the herd.

Consequence

Although the precise impact of virus latency was only recognized during the latest 15 years (Blaskovic *et al.*, 1970, Sabo and Rajcani, 1976, Gutekunst, 1979, Beran *et al.*, 1980, Rziha *et al.*, 1982), from the beginning of our control programme the recovered pigs and infected herds were considered being a virus reservoir and excluded from trade. The restriction in swine trade from infected herds is the most important determining factor to minimize further virus spread.

Third determining factor

Immunisations, carried out with either live or inactivated vaccines, do not modify an already established latency of field virus and do not absolutely prevent the adsorption, penetration and multiplication of virus at the natural primary sites of virus replication (Blaskovic *et al.*, 1970). Consequently, new latent virus carriers can arise without showing clinical signs, because immunisation usually will protect the pig against development of clinical signs.

Consequence

All vaccinated herds were, with respect to trade of pigs, assessed as infected herds, as long as it was not proven, that ADV-seropositive pigs were no longer present. Because antibodies induced by vaccination could not be differentiated from those induced by infection, in principle, only "metaphylactic" vaccination was carried out. Thus, only herds where AD was diagnosed were vaccinated. This metaphylactic vaccination was performed in all herds, except in those cleaned-up by test and removal, selection procedures or stamping-out measures. No regulations were therefore necessary for herds free of infections, and if in these free herds antibodies were found it was evidence of infection. Vaccination of all infected herds will considerably reduce virus replication, both by enhancing the threshold of infectivity and by reduction of virus replication in animals that still became infected. Consequently, the "infection pressure" in an area is strongly diminished.

The fourth determining factor

The course of infection in pig herds is basically dependent on the size of the herd (number of pigs), the number of pigs per square meter, which determines the intensity of contact among pigs, and the extent of movement of pigs within a herd as well as introductions from outside. In smaller, closed herds an infection often will result in a percentage of infected animals below 30%, and with time few additional animals will encounter infection. Reactivation of viurs latency can sometimes initiate recrudescence of infection. On the other hand, in very large pig herds with thousands of sows or over 10,000 fatteners, due to the high intensity of contacts between pigs, the replacements of pigs and the frequent introductions of new pigs, there is a continuous circulation leading to newly infected pigs, also when more than 90% of the herd is seropositive. When an acute primary infection takes place in such an enormous herd, virus is generated to such a high level, that there is an additional danger of airborne spread from the herd (Donaldson *et al.*, 1983, Gloster *et al.*, 1984, Kaaden, 1985).

Consequence

These features must certainly be taken into account when herds are cleaned-up. In small herds, a herd clean-up frequently succeeded by identifying, selecting and removing of reagents, supported by general hygienic measures and re-examination of individual animals (Kretzschmar, 1970). In very large herds, even intensive vaccination is no guarantee that the infection can be completely suppressed, so that a complete depopulation-repopulation strategy is inevitable. With moderately-sized herds the infection can be arrested by several premise-based measures, particulary stopping the purchase and internal movement of pigs in combination with consistent vaccination and a gradual replacement of pigs. In addition, hygienic measures are taken to restrict indirect transmission by low levels of residual virus.

AD shows, when compared to other infectious diseases, some features that facilitate the eradication of the virus.

1. The chance of virus transmission, by passive transfer through vectors, is very low.

2. Irrespective of the broad natural host spectrum of the virus, the infection will disappear when it has been eradicated from swine. Although in rats the infection can be maintained for a certain period, particularly because they eat the diseased or dead rats, the infection eventually will "die out" in rat populations, because they virtually all die from AD.

Virus transmission among other species can also incidentally take place.

3. The piglets from seropositive sows are free of virus after disappearance of maternal antibodies and when grown in isolation can be used for replacing seropositive sows.

4. Immunotolerance is no disturbing factor in eradication. Pigs that survived the infection react uniformly with the formation of antibodies.

5. The diagnosis, in particular the serological diagnosis, can be made fast, is simple to perform, has a high specificity and sensitivity and is reliable. Therefore, mass serological screenings, which are required in an eradication programme, can be performed.

6. The 24 hour virus neutralization test with an early microscopic reading as well as the solid-phase ELISA are equally well suitable for diagnosis of the individual animal. For evaluating the herd situation with random sampling a more simple neutralisation test in mictrotitre plates or tubes will do.

Some other aspects that we encountered during the eradication scheme should be mentioned. Although they are not essential, they anyway improve the economical efficacy and security.

1. In enzootically infected areas the spread of infection is not seldom by feeding garbage, when it is not adequately heated.

2. An effective rat control programme is of value in the control of AD. Rats often prefer to build nests in pig stables (Schuster, 1984). ADV can circulate independently in rat populations for some weeks. As a consequence, infected rats may play a role in transmission of the virus from one herd to another. Norway rats normally swarm off in groups to other places, when the population exceeds a certain limit or when the food situation is bad, and other conditions grow worse, for instance in connection with removing of swine herds. Large swine herds should, therefore, be kept free of rats.

3. In feral pigs the pathogenesis of the infection is similar to that in domestic pigs. In wooded areas with a high density of feral pigs one should bear in mind the danger of persistence of ADV in the feral pig population.

PROGRESS OF THE ERADICATION PROGRAMME IN THE GERMAN DEMOCRATIC REPUBLIC

The success of an eradication programme for an infectious disease is determined by the ability to 1) restrict the spread of the infection in a certain area, 2) eliminate the causative agent in the infected herd.

The quality and rightness of eradication schemes are to be evaluated on the basis of 2 parameters:

1. The number of new cases in a certain period, expressed as a percentage of

the number of cases in the beginning of that period.

2. The number of cleared herds in comparison with the original situation and new cases.

The first parameter is an indication of the "infection pressure" in a certain region or country, the second of the intensity of the cleaning-up procedures.

Table 1 shows the development of these parameters in our Magdeburg District (Kretzschmar, 1987). It is shown, that in the second time period the mere

TABLE 1 Results of clean-up procedures and development of the regional "infection pressure" of Aujeszky's disease in a district related to the clean-up strategies

Period	Number of infected herds				Average yearly regional "infection pressure" in % = no. of new cases/no. of infected herds at the beginning of the year
	at start	at end	new	cleared	
1960-1964 Notifying clinical outbreaks and short-term prohibition of trade	1	58	60	3	110
1965-1969 Start of nationwide serological survey and long-term prohibition of trade of infected herds	58	93	178	143	38
1970-1976 Increased vaccination of infected herds to prepare their clearing	93	16	38	115	10
1977-1982 As in period 1970-1976; concentration of pigs into fewer herds	16	10	30	36	69
1983-1985 Vaccination and stamping-out within a few months	10	0	1	11	17

identification of all infected herds and their prohibition to enter trade, reduced the regional "infection pressure" from 110 to 38. In the third period there is a decrease from 38 to 10, partially due to the metaphylactic vaccination in infected herds, which are not allowed to trade pigs with free herds. The fourth period is characterized by a stagnation, associated with a concentration of pigs into fewer herds. Although the absolute number of infected herds was low, the successful clean-ups were almost neutralized by the new cases; the "infection pressure" was considerably increased. It was not until the fifth time period when the eradication was definitely accomplished. In this period stamping out procedures were predominantly followed. A part of the herds was vaccinated, fattened and moved to slaughter. These procedures comprised a total of approximately 250,000 pigs.

In our eradication scheme a consistent and "lückenlos" ("holeless") vaccination was used in infected herds for several years, until a complete new generation of breeding pigs had been built up. Not until vaccination was discontinued it was possible to examine in newly introduced pigs whether field virus had been disappeared from the herd. In most instances, the field virus was no longer present. In some herds, however, a new infection began and thus destroyed long-term attempts to clean-up herds; as a consequence a new danger for the environment arose. At present, such situations can be prevented, if a genetically deleted vaccine virus (Lomniczi *et al.*, 1984, Gielkens *et al.*, 1985) is employed, which enables the differentiation between antibodies induced by vaccination and by infection (Van Oirschot *et al.*, 1986).

At present, we will not generally decline the use of live vaccines. We have favourable experiences with the K-61 strain (Bartha, 1961). We will require, however, that the vaccine used will not establish latency in pigs. The K-61 strain seems to meet this requirement. With regard to eradication a prerequisite is the "holeless" immunisation of the entire herd with revaccinations for periods longer than generation period in breeding herds, or a fattening period in fattening herds. Attempts, to reduce the time of the entire herd vaccination, have always failed, because reactivation of a latent infection is then the beginning of a recrudescent infection.

EPIZOOTIOLOGICAL EXPERIENCES SINCE THE ERADICATION OF AD FROM THE GERMAN DEMOCRATIC REPUBLIC

Since the eradication of AD in 1985, 4 small clinical outbreaks were diagnosed close to the border with the enzootically infected Federal Republic of Germany. One infected herd, in the inland, was identified by serological examination. All herds were cleaned-up by stamping-out in some weeks. In a clinical outbreak in our Magdeburg District the virus was clearly introduced by stray rats. There was a massive movement of diseased rats, of which a considerable number died, into a pig premise, followed by signs of disease among piglets about 2 weeks later. Virus was isolated from these piglets. Then a diseased rat was killed and it was found to harbour ADV in its blood. Among 48 rats that were killed in the next week, virus was isolated from 1 rat. Furthermore, virus was isolated from a polecat (Putorius putorius), known to be a rat eater, which was found dead on the premise.

In the outbreak in the inland there had probably been contact with feral pigs. The percentage of seropositive feral pigs was highest in the border area with an enzootically infected neighbouring country and lowered as one proceeded into the direction of the infected area.

The yearly serological screening programme of the entire national swine population is to be continued.

REFERENCES

Bartha, A. 1961. Experiments to reduce the virulence of Aujeszky's virus. Magy. Allartorv. Lap. **16,** 42-45.

Blaskovic, D., Sabo, A. and Rajcani, J. 1970. Experimentelle Pathogenese der Aujeszkyschen Krankheit beim Ferkel. Arch. Exp. Vet. Med., **24,** 9-27.

Beran, G.W., Davies, E.B., Arambulo, P.V., Will, L.A., Hill, H.T., and Rock, D.L. 1980. Persistence of pseudorabies virus in infected swine. J. Am. Vet. Med. Ass., **176,** 998-1000.

Donaldson, A.I., Wardley, R.C., Martin, S., and Ferris, N.P. 1983. Experimental Aujeszky's disease in pigs: excretion, survival and transmission of the virus. Vet. Rec., **113,** 490-494.

Gielkens, A.L.J., Van Oirschot, J.T. and Berns, A.J.M. 1985. Genome differences among field isolates and vaccine strains of pseudorabies virus. J. Gen. Virol., **66,** 69-82.

Gloster, J., Donaldson, A.I. and Hough, M.N. 1984. Analysis of a series of outbreaks of Aujeszky's disease in Yorkshire in 1981-1982. The possibility of airborne disease spread. Vet. Rec., **114,** 234-239.

Gutekunst, D.E. 1979. Latent pseudorabies virus infection in swine detected by RNA-DNA hybridization. Am. J. Vet. Res. **40,** 1568-1572.

Kaaden, O.R. 1985. Luft als Vektor viraler Krankheitserreger. Tierärztl. Umschau, **40,** 4-10.

Kretzschmar, Ch. 1970. Die Aujeszkysche Krankheit. VEB Gustav Fischer Verlag, Jena.

Kretzschmar, Ch. 1973. Zum Wert der aktiven Immunisiering mit Lebendimpfstoff bei der Sanierung der Bestände von Aujeszkyscher Krankheit. Mh. Vet. Med., **28,** 927-931.

Kretzschmar, Ch. 1987. Erfahrungen, Wege und Ergebnisse im historischen Ablauf der Bekämpfung der Aujeszkyschen Krankheit bis zu ihrer Tilgung in der DDR im Jahre 1985. Mh. Vet. Med. **42,** 155-158.

Lomniczi, B., Blankenship, M.L., Ben-Porat, T. 1984. Deletions in the genomes of pseudorabies virus vaccine strains and existence of four isomers of the genomes. J. Virol., **49,** 970-979.

Rziha, H.J., Döller, P.C., Wittmann, G. 1982. Detection of Aujeszky's disease virus and viral DNA in tissues of latently infected pigs. Curr. top. Vet. Med. Ani. Sci., **17,** 205-210. In: CEC Seminar on "Aujeszky's disease" (G. Wittmann and S.A. Hall, Eds). (Martinus Nijhoff, The Hague).

Sabo, A. and Rajcani, J. 1976. Latent pseudorabies infection in pigs. Acta Virol., **20,** 208-214.

Schuster, W. 1984. Untersuchungen zum Vorkommen der Haus- und Wanderratte im Bezirk Magdeburg und Darstellung eines Modells zu ihrer Bekämpfung. Diss. rer. nat. Päd. Hochsch. Potsdam.

Van Oirschot, J.T., Rziha, H.J., Moonen, P.J.L.M., Pol, J.M.A. and Van Zaane, D. 1986. Differentiation of serum antibodies from pigs vaccinated or infected with Aujeszky's disease virus by a competitive enzyme immunoassay. J. Gen. Virol., **67,** 1179-1182.

SUMMARY

In this session, 8 speakers presented information on the Aujeszky's disease (AD) situation and the measures taken or not taken in their respective countries. A total of 8 nations was represented.

Pensaert (Belgium) presented the results of a study related to the replication of AD virus (ADV) in the respiratory tract of susceptible and immune pigs. Pigs 1 month immune after a previous infection, allow virus replication in their deeper air pathways upon intracheal challenge. Free bronchio-alveolar cells remain susceptible and probably become rather easily infected also in strongly immune animals. They can carry the virus to the alveoli which become infected by cell to cell contact. Control by vaccination may, therefore, be a rather difficult goal to achieve in densely populated regions where the risk of infection in vaccinated animals remains high.

The control and eradication of ADV in Denmark was discussed by Andersen who pointed out taht airborne spread of the virulent virus from a neighbouring country was the only cause of new disease outbreaks in Denmark in 1987. He, therefore, made a strong appeal for international cooperation in the control of AD and indicated the urgency with which measures should be taken in all member states of the European Community (EC).

Taylor (England) reported on the successful control program in his country and found that movement of subclinically infected pigs prior to, during or shortly after an outbreak is the main problem during the last stages of the eradication process; he found airborne infections to be of minor importance.

Thawley (USA) updated the events occurring in the control of AD in the USA where programs vary from vaccination to test and removal, to offspring segregation, to depopulation and repopulation. Control programs are different in different states. Apparently, AD still has a rather mild course in the USA.

Wittmann (FRG) gave a short history on the situation of AD in his country and the poor success encountered in the control in the past. He discussed the new proposals made in 1987 in which an intensive vaccination program with deleted vaccines (gI-negative), even though very costly, is set forward as a first step towards eradication.

Vannier (France) presented the favourable results of the control program encountered in some departments but pointed toward the high rate of infection observed in regions with high density swine populations. Based on the experience in Brittany, he warned the audience not to be too optimistic with regard to control of AD by intensive vaccination in dense swine populations in which the virus in

J. T. van Oirschot (ed.), Vaccination and Control of Aujeszky's Disease, 249–250.

enzootic.

Papadopoulos (Greece) reported on AD in his country and stressed that outbreaks in Greece have been "imported" with infected swine from other member states. He pleaded for a common strategy in all EC countries, which should take the risk away for importing countries.

McCullough (Northern Ireland) reported on the AD situation in his country in which vaccination with an attenuated vaccine is allowed but in which eradication in encouraged by registration of AD free herds. He presented some experiments in which the relationship was shown between virulence of virus strains and the rate of excretion and the ability to spread within a swine population.

Kretzschmar (DDR) did not present his paper at the seminar, but it was considered worthwile to insert experiences on the control of AD in the DDR into the proceedings.

In general terms, eradication by slaughter is the most straightforward method for control of AD, but it is only feasible in countries with a favourable epizootiologic situation. In dense swine populations, there is little choice and intensive vaccination with the use of deleted vaccines, in which vaccinated animals can be differentiated from infected ones, is set forward. Common strategies should be used in the different EC member states with regard to the measures taken, vaccine types used and tests applied for differentiation.

There is a definite need for comparative evaluation tests on vaccines, to be carried out on an international basis with the purpose to obtain clear viewpoints on whether (some) deletions are harmful or not for the immunogenicity of vaccine strains. In the light of eradication, evaluation of vaccines should certainly directed towards epizootiological aspects, i.e. which vaccine or vaccination schedule is optimal to prevent infection with virulent virus in vaccinated pigs or, if not able to prevent, which is the most efficient in reducing virulent virus replication and excretion when vaccinated pigs become infected. Several participants were of the opinion that the evaluation tests should be carried out objectively and urgently and as a cooperative project beween EC member states.

CONCLUDING REMARKS

Aujeszky's disease (AD), caused by a herpesvirus, is one of the most important virus diseases affecting today's pig industry. Eradication of Aujeszky's disease virus (ADV) would be a great economic benefit troughout the world.

The glycoproteins of ADV play an important role in determining the virulence and immunogenicity of the virus. The major glycoproteins have been identified, characterized, and mapped on the genome, and their genes have been sequenced. The virus has several glycoproteins that are not required for replication of the virus in cell cultures and in pigs. Some of the functions of these nonessential glycoproteins have been elucidated. The structural nonessential glycoproteins gI, gp63, and gIII are determinants of virulence, but the nonstructural gX glycoprotein is not. Glycoprotein gIII is involved in virus adsorption to the cell, and gIII as well as gI play a role in virus release from the cell. Glycoprotein gIII appears to be more important in eliciting an immune response to the virus than gI, gp63, or gX.

Deletion mutant viruses that do not express gI, or gX, or gIII have recently been constructed. In addition, they have been rendered thymidine kinase negative. These deletion mutants can be used as vaccine viruses; their genomic structure being better characterized than that of conventionally prepared, modified-live vaccines.

Many ADV vaccines, conventionally prepared as well as genetically engineered, are used for pigs. Many reports on efficacy of these vaccines have been published, but, due to widely varying test conditions, it is difficult, if not impossible, to identify the most efficacious vaccine(s).

Because of these variances, the efficacy of vaccines should be evaluated, preferably in one experiment, in the laboratory under strictly standardized conditions. Criteria for efficacy are the vaccine's ability to prevent or reduce: 1) mortality, 2) weight loss, 3) fever, and 4) shedding of challenge virus. Ideally, the efficacy of vaccines would be determined by vaccinating and then challenging seronegative pigs, and pigs with maternal antibodies, and by challenging unvaccinated piglets born from vaccinated sows. Each experiment includes seronegative control pigs.

Although pig producers are often concerned primarily with the vaccine's ability to protect against clinical disease, with regard to control of ADV more important is the ability of the vaccine to 1) reduce shedding of challenge virus, 2) enhance the threshold of infectivity, and 3) prevent the establishment of latency. Vaccination generally does not prevent pigs from becoming infected after challenge, and consequently the challenge virus may remain latent.

J. T. van Oirschot (ed.), Vaccination and Control of Aujeszky's Disease, 251–253.

LIST OF PARTICIPANTS

Belgium

Dr. G. Florent, Smith-Kline RIT, Rue de l'Institut 89, B-1330 Rixensart
Dr. F. Koenen, Nationaal Instituut voor Diergeneeskundig Onderzoek, Groeselenberg 99, B-1180 Brussels
Dr. C. Miry, Fakulteit Diergeneeskunde, Laboratorium voor Virologie, Casinoplein 24, B-9000 Gent
Dr. C. Muelenaere, Fakulteit Diergeneeskunde, Laboratorium voor Virologie, Casinoplein 24, B-9000 Gent
Prof. Dr. M. Pensaert, Fakulteit Diergeneeskunde, Laboratorium voor Virologie, Casinoplein 24, B-9000 Gent

Denmark

Dr. J.B. Andersen, The Veterinary Directorate, 21 Frederiksgade, DK-1265 Copenhagen K
Dr. L.S. Christensen, State Veterinary Institute for Veterinary Research, Lindholm, DK-4771 Kalvehave
Dr. P. Have, State Veterinary Institute for Veterinary Research, Lindholm DK-4771 Kalvehave

Federal Republic of Germany

P.B. Lebeau, Agritech Systems GmbH, Hindenburgstrasse 42, D-6500 Mainz 1
Dr. T.C. Mettenleiter, Bundesforschungsanstalt für Viruskrankheiten der Tiere, Paul Ehrlichstrasse 28, D-7400 Tübingen
Dr. H.J. Rziha, Bundesforschungsanstalt für Viruskrankheiten der Tiere, Paul Ehrlichstrasse 28, D-7400 Tübingen
Prof. Dr. G. Wittmann, Bundesforschungsanstalt für Viruskrankheiten der Tiere, Paul Ehrlichstrasse 28, D-7400 Tübingen

France

Dr. G. Chappuis, IFFA Mérieux, 254 rue Marcel Mérieux, F-69007 Lyon
Dr. M. Eloit, Ecole Nationale Vétérinaire d'Alfort, 7 Avenue du Général de Gaulle, F-94704 Maisons-Alfort Cedex
Dr. A. Jestin, Station de Pathologie Porcine, B.P. no 9, F-22440 Ploufragan
Prof. Dr. B. Toma, Ecole Nationale Vétérinaire d'Alfort, 7 Avenue du Général de Gaulle, F-94704 Maisons-Alfort Cedex
Dr. J. Vandeputte, IFFA Mérieux, 254 rue Marcel Mérieux, F-69007 Lyon
Dr. P. Vannier, Station de Pathologie Porcine, B.P. no 9, F-22440 Ploufragan

Greece

Prof. Dr. O. Papadopoulos, Aristotelian University, Faculty of Veterinary Medicine, Departement of Microbiology and, Infectious Diseases, G-54006 Thessaloniki

Hungary

Dr. B. Lomniczi, Veterinary Medical Research Institute, Hungarian Academy of Sciences, P.O.B. 18, H-1581 Budapest

Ireland

Dr. P.J. O'Connor, Veterinary Research Laboratory, Abbotstown, Castleknock, Dublin

Italy

Dr. M. Amadori, Istituto zooprofilattico, Via Bianchi 7, I-25100 Brescia

The Netherlands

Dr. A.L.J. Gielkens, Centraal Diergeneeskundig Instituut, Houtribweg 39, 8221 RA Lelystad
Dr. C.E. Jacobs, Centraal Diergeneeskundig Instituut, Edelhertweg 15, 8219 PH Lelystad
Dr. A.F.C. Kuiper, Duphar BV, PO Box 2, 1380 AA Weesp
Dr. T.G. Kimman, Centraal Diergeneeskundig Instituut, Houtribweg 39, 8221 RA Lelystad
Dr. D. Lütticken, Intervet International BV, PO Box 31, 5830 AA Boxmeer
Dr. J.T. van Oirschot, Centraal Diergeneeskundig Instituut, Edelhertweg 15,8219 PH Lelystad
Dr. P.C. van der Valk, Ministry of Agriculture and Fisheries, Bezuidenhoutseweg 73, 2500 EK 's-Gravenhage

Portugal

Dr. A.P.M. Valadares, Laboratorio Nacional de, Investigacao Veterinaria, Est. de Benfica 701, P-1500 Lisboa

Spain

Dr. P. Carmenes, Departemento Patalogia Animal: Sanidad Animal, Facultad de Veterinaria, Campus de la Vegezana, S-24007 Léon
Dr. J. Plana Duran, Laboratorios Sobrino s.a., S-17813 Vall de Bianya (Gerona)

United Kingdom

Dr. S.J. McCullough, Veterinary Research Laboratories, Stormont , Belfast, BT4 3SD

Dr. K. Taylor, Veterinary Services, Government Building, Hookrise South, Tolworth, Surbiton, Surrey KT6 7NF

United States of America

Prof. Dr. T. Ben-Porat, Vanderbilt University, School of Medicine, Department of Microbiology, Nashville TN 37232

Prof. Dr. S. Kit, Baylor College of Medicine, Department of Virology and Epidemiology, Division of Biochemical Virology, Houston TX 77030

Dr. R.D. MacDonald, Syntro Corporation, 10655 Sorrento Valley Road, San Diego CA 92121

Dr. R.B. Morrison, University of Minnesota, Department of Large Animal Clinical Sciences, College of Veterinary Medicine, 225 Veterinary Teaching Hospitals, 1365 Gortner Avenue, St. Paul, Minnesota 55108

Dr. L.E. Post, The Upjohn Company, Kalamazoo, Michigan 49001

Prof. Dr. D.G. Thawley, University of Minnesota, Department of Large Animal Clinical Sciences, College of Veterinary Medicine, 225 Veterinary Teaching Hospitals, 1365 Gortner Avenue, St. Paul, Minnesota 55108

Dr. J.D. Todd, Syntrovet, 9669 Lackman Road, Lenexa, Kansas 66219

Dr. R.C. Wardley, The Upjohn Company, Kalamazoo, Michigan 49001

Yugoslavia

Dr. V. Rukavina, Export Department, PLIVA, I.L. Ribara 89, 41001 Zagreb

Printed in the United States
136854LV00003B/34/A

9 780792 301844